ANXIETY AND DEPRESSION INFORMATION FOR TEENS FIRST EDITION

ANXIETY AND DEPRESSION INFORMATION FOR TEENS FIRST EDITION

Health Tips about Mental-Health Disorders, Types, Diagnosis, and Treatment of Anxiety and Depression

Including Facts about the Protective Factors and Mental-Health Support, Mental-Health Literacy, and Living with Mental-Health Condition

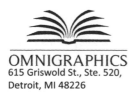

OMNIGRAPHICS
615 Griswold St., Ste. 520,
Detroit, MI 48226

Bibliographic Note

Because this page cannot legibly accommodate all the copyright notices, the Bibliographic Note portion of the Preface constitutes an extension of the copyright notice.

* * *

OMNIGRAPHICS

Kevin Hayes, *Managing Editor*

* * *

Library of Congress Cataloging-in-Publication Data

Names: Hayes, Kevin (Editor of health information), editor.

Title: Anxiety and depression information for teens: basic health information on anxiety and depression in teens and its various types, the causes, risk factors, diagnosis, treatments, and coping methods including information about managing anxiety and depression with the help of family, friends, pets, and relaxation techniques / edited by Kevin Hayes.

Description: First edition. | Detroit, MI: Omnigraphics, Inc., 2020. | Series: Teen health series | Includes index. | Audience: Ages 13 | Audience: Grades 7-9 | Summary: "Provides basic health information on anxiety and depression in teens and its various types, causes, risk factors, diagnosis, treatments, and coping methods. Includes an index, and a directory of organizations for additional help and information"-- Provided by publisher.

Identifiers: LCCN 2020027663 (print) | LCCN 2020027664 (ebook) | ISBN 9780780818200 (library binding) | ISBN 9780780818217 (ebook)

Subjects: LCSH: Anxiety in adolescence--Juvenile literature. | Depression in adolescence--Juvenile literature.

Classification: LCC RJ506.A58 A57 2020 (print) | LCC RJ506.A58 (ebook) | DDC 616.85/2700835--dc23

LC record available at https://lccn.loc.gov/2020027663

LC ebook record available at https://lccn.loc.gov/2020027664

TABLE OF CONTENTS

Part 3 | Diagnosis and Treatment for Anxiety and Depression

Part 4 | Strengthening Protective Factors and Mental-Health Support

Part 5 | Living with a Mental-Health Condition

Part 6 | If You Need More Help or Information

PREFACE

About This Book

People affected by anxiety suffer from intense and uncontrollable feelings of anxiety, fear, worry, and/or panic. When a person is in a sad mood for a prolonged period of time and it interferes with their daily normal activities she or he might be depressed which sometimes might be due to anxiety. Some symptoms of anxiety and depression are feeling sad and anxious often, losing interest in one's favorite activity, feeling easily irritated or frustrated, etc. According to the Centers for Disease Control and Prevention (CDC), an estimated 19.1 percent of U.S. adults had at least one of the anxiety disorders in 2003. Similarly, in 2017, about 11 million U.S. adults 18 years of age or older had at least one major depressive episode.

Anxiety and Depression Information for Teens, First Edition offers an insight into adolescent mental health, the basics of decoding the teen brain and provides basic information on anxiety and depression. It explains the major types of anxiety such as generalized anxiety disorder (GAD), separation anxiety disorder (SAD), selective mutism (SM), specific phobias, agoraphobia, social anxiety disorder (SAD), panic disorder (PD), etc. It gives in-depth information about diagnosis and treatment options for anxiety and depression. It highlights how to manage anxiety and depression with the help of therapies and technology. There is also information on coping with protective and promotive factors and mental-health support. It offers helpful information on unique issues in emotional and social development in adolescence, the importance of school connectedness, positive youth development for sexual minorities, dealing with bullying, learning to resist peer pressure, healthy ways to cope with stress, handling suicidal thoughts and increasing mental-health literacy, help-seeking attitudes, and reducing stigma. It provides useful information on how to access mental-health services, health insurance coverage, school-based support, and mental healthcare during COVID-19 for treating mental health in teens. Controlling vape cravings, cutting back on caffeine, academic accommodations for students with psychiatric disability, and workplace accommodations for youth with mental-health needs are also covered in this book. A directory of organizations that help people with anxiety, depression, and other mental-health concerns is also included.

How to Use This Book

This book is divided into parts and chapters. Parts focus on broad areas of interest; chapters are devoted to single topics within a part.

Part 1: Understanding Mental-Health Disorders explains about the adolescent mental health and the basics of decoding the teen brain. It provides information on mental health in teens, some common mental-health myths, and mental-health related challenges faced by the teens. It also highlights risk and protective factors and presents information on mental-health promotion and prevention.

Part 2: Major Types of Anxiety Disorders and Depression describes the major types of anxiety and depression seen in teens. It elaborates about various anxiety disorders such as generalized anxiety disorder (GAD), separation anxiety disorder (SAD), selective mutism (SM), specific phobias, agoraphobia, social anxiety disorder (SAD), and panic disorder (PD) and explains how hoarding is a major form of anxiety disorder. It also covers information on different depressive disorders such as disruptive mood dysregulation disorder (DMDD), major depressive disorder (MDD), persistent depressive disorder (dysthymic disorder), premenstrual dysphoric disorder, and substance-induced depressive and anxiety disorder.

Part 3: Diagnosis and Treatment of Anxiety Disorders and Depression provides information on the diagnosis and treatment of anxiety disorders and depression along with a focus on treatment options and therapy for anxiety. Useful details are given on how exposure therapy, play and creative art therapy, family therapy, and complementary approaches are treatments for anxiety and depression and also for comorbid disorders. The part closes with an outline of how the latest technologies have improved the future of mental-health treatments.

Part 4: Strengthening Protective Factors and Mental-Health Support provides guidance on how anxiety and depression can be managed by strengthening protective factors and mental-health support. It offers helpful information on unique issues in emotional and social development in adolescence, protective and promotive factors, the importance of school connectedness, positive youth development for sexual minorities, dealing with bullying, learning to resist peer pressure, healthy ways to cope with stress, handling suicidal thoughts and increasing mental-health literacy, help-seeking attitudes, and reducing stigma.

Part 5: Living with a Mental-Health Condition explains how it is like to live with anxiety and how to face mental-health issues. It provides useful information on how to access mental-health services, health insurance coverage, school-based support, along with tips for good mental health during COVID-19 situation. It discusses how teens may think about using vape and caffeine as an outlet for anxiety and depression and provide tips on how to prevent or quit them. It also covers academic accommodations for students with psychiatric disability and workplace accommodations for youth with mental health.

Part 6: If You Need More Information provides a list of government and private organizations that provide help and support for people with anxiety, depression, and other mental-health concerns.

Bibliographic Note

This volume contains documents and excerpts from publications issued by the following U.S. government agencies: Agency for Healthcare Research and Quality (AHRQ); Centers for Disease Control and Prevention (CDC); Centers for Medicare & Medicaid Services (CMS); Child Welfare Information Gateway; National Center for Complementary and Integrative Health (NCCIH); National Council on Disability (NCD); National Institute of Diabetes and Digestive and Kidney Diseases (NIDDK); National Institute of Mental Health (NIMH); National Institute on Drug Abuse (NIDA); National Institute on Drug Abuse (NIDA) for Teens; National Institute on Minority Health and Health Disparities (NIMHD); National Institutes of Health (NIH); *NIH News in Health*; Office of Adolescent Health (OAH); Office of Disability Employment Policy (ODEP); Substance Abuse and Mental Health Services Administration (SAMHSA); U.S. Department of Health and Human Services (HHS); U.S. Department of Veterans Affairs (VA); U.S. Food and Drug Administration (FDA); and Youth.gov.

It may also contain original material produced by Omnigraphics and reviewed by medical consultants.

The photograph on the front cover is © Diego Cervo/Shutterstock.

Medical Review

Omnigraphics contracts with a team of qualified, senior medical professionals who serve as medical consultants for the *Teen Health Series*. As necessary, medical consultants review reprinted and originally written material for currency and accuracy. Citations including the phrase "Reviewed (month, year)" indicate material reviewed by this team. Medical consultation services are provided to the *Teen Health Series* editors by:

Dr. Vijayalakshmi, MBBS, DGO, MD
Dr. Senthil Selvan, MBBS, DCH, MD
Dr. K. Sivanandham, MBBS, DCH, MS (Research), PhD

About The *Teen Health Series*

At the request of librarians serving today's teens and young adults, the *Teen Health Series* was developed as a specially focused set of volumes within Omnigraphics' *Health Reference Series*. Each volume deals comprehensively with a topic selected according to the needs and interests of people in middle school and high school. Teens seeking preventive guidance, information about disease warning signs, medical statistics, and risk factors for health problems will find answers to their questions in the *Teen Health Series*. The *Series*, however, is not intended to serve as a tool for diagnosing illness, in prescribing treatments, or as a substitute for the physician–patient relationship. All people concerned about medical symptoms or the possibility of disease are encouraged to seek professional care from an appropriate healthcare provider.

If there is a topic you would like to see addressed in a future volume of the *Teen Health Series*, please write to:

Managing Editor
Teen Health Series
Omnigraphics
615 Griswold St., Ste. 520
Detroit, MI 48226

A Note About Spelling And Style

Teen Health Series editors use *Stedman's Medical Dictionary* as an authority for questions related to the spelling of medical terms and *The Chicago Manual of Style* for questions related to grammatical structures, punctuation, and other editorial concerns. Consistent adherence is not always possible, however, because the individual volumes within the *Series* include many documents from a wide variety of different producers and copyright holders, and the editor's primary goal is to present material from each source as accurately as is possible following the terms specified by each document's producer. This sometimes means that information in different chapters may follow other guidelines and alternate spelling authorities. For example, occasionally a copyright holder may require that eponymous terms be shown in possessive forms (Crohn's disease vs. Crohn disease) or that British spelling norms be retained (leukaemia vs. leukemia).

PART 1 | UNDERSTANDING MENTAL-HEALTH DISORDERS

CHAPTER 1
ADOLESCENT MENTAL HEALTH

About This Chapter: Text in this chapter begins with excerpts from "Adolescent Mental Health Basics,"
Office of Adolescent Health (OAH), U.S. Department of Health and Human Services (HHS), May 14,
2020; Text under the heading "Common Mental Health Warning Signs" is excerpted from "Common
Mental Health Warning Signs," Office of Adolescent Health (OAH), U.S. Department of Health and Human
Services (HHS), January 15, 2019.

Some adolescents will experience a serious mental-health disorder at some point in their life, and problems with mental health can start early in life. The good news is that promoting positive mental health can prevent some problems from starting. For young people who already have mental-health disorders, early intervention and treatment can help lessen the impact on their lives.

Impact of Mental-Health Problems in Adolescence

It is a normal part of development for teens to experience a wide range of emotions. It is typical, for instance, for teens to feel anxious about school or friendships, or to experience a period of depression following the death of a close friend or family member. Mental-health disorders, however, are characterized by persistent symptoms that affect how a young person feels, thinks, and acts. Mental-health disorders also can interfere with regular activities and daily functioning, such as relationships, schoolwork, sleeping, and eating.

Important mental-health habits—including coping, resilience, and good judgement—help adolescents to achieve overall well-being and set the stage for positive mental health in adulthood. Mood swings are common during adolescence. However, some adolescents will experience a serious mental-health disorder, such as depression and/or anxiety disorders, at some point in their life. Friends and family can watch for warning signs of mental disorders and urge young people to get help. Effective treatments exist and may involve a combination of psychotherapy and medication. Unfortunately, less than half of adolescents with psychiatric disorders receive any kind of treatment.

Depression is the most common mental-health disorder, affecting nearly one in eight adolescents and young adults each year. Adolescents who experience symptoms of depression most of the day, nearly every day, for at least two weeks in the year are having a major depressive episode. The number of adolescents who experienced major depressive episodes increased by nearly a third from 2005 to 2014.

When left untreated, mental-health disorders can lead to serious—even life-threatening—consequences. Depression, other mental-health disorders, and substance use disorders are major risk factors for suicide. Suicide is the second leading cause of death for 15- to 24-year-olds. In 2013 and 2014, children ages 10 to 14 were more likely to die from suicide than in a motor vehicle accident. Any concerns that family members or healthcare providers have about an adolescent's mental health should be promptly addressed.

Common Mental-Health Warning Signs

Mental health is not simply the presence or absence of symptoms. Mental health includes generally feeling and functioning well and resiliently when faced with setbacks. Adolescents may have different symptoms than adults with the same mental-health disorder and symptoms may vary from person to person. Some adolescents only experience one or two symptoms while others experience more. Furthermore, adolescents may experience symptoms only once or infrequently, in which case they may be just experiencing emotions that are common at this age. These variations can make identification and diagnosis of mental-health disorders challenging. According to the National Institute of Mental Health (NIMH) (www.nimh.nih.gov/health/topics/child-and-adolescent-mental-health/index.shtml), a child or teen might need help if they:

- Often feel very angry or very worried
- Have difficulty sleeping or eating
- Lose interest in activities that they used to enjoy
- Isolate themselves and avoid social interactions
- Feel grief for a long time after a loss or death
- Use alcohol, tobacco, or other drugs
- Obsessively exercise, diet, and/or binge eat
- Hurt other people or destroy property
- Have low or no energy
- Feel like they cannot control their emotions
- Have thoughts of suicide
- Harm themselves (e.g., burning or cutting their skin)
- Think their mind is being controlled or is out of control
- Hear voices

If you observe a teen experiencing these symptoms and need to seek help, consult your healthcare provider or mental-health professional. In crisis or life-threatening situations, call 911, contact the National Suicide Prevention Lifeline (suicidepreventionlifeline.org), or go to your nearest hospital emergency room. Visit NIMH's Help for Mental Illness (www.nimh.nih.gov/health/find-help/index.shtml) page for more details and to identify treatment options in your area.

CHAPTER 2
DECODING THE TEEN BRAIN

About This Chapter: This chapter includes text excerpted from "The Teen Brain: 7 Things to Know,"
National Institute of Mental Health (NIMH), 2020.

Did you know that big and important changes are happening in the brain during adolescence? Here are 7 things to know about the teen brain:

The Brain Reaches Its Biggest Size in Early Adolescence

For girls, the brain reaches its biggest size around 11 years old. For boys, the brain reaches its biggest size around age 14. But, this difference does not mean either boys or girls are smarter than one another!

The Brain Continues to Mature Even after It Is Done Growing

Though the brain may be done growing in size, it does not finish developing and maturing until the mid- to late-20s. The front part of the brain, called the "prefrontal cortex," is one of the last brain regions to mature. This area is responsible for skills such as planning, prioritizing, and controlling impulses. Because these skills are still developing, teens are more likely to engage in risky behaviors without considering the potential results of their decisions.

The Teen Brain Is Ready to Learn and Adapt

The teen brain has lots of plasticity, which means it can change, adapt, and respond to its environment. Challenging academics or mental activities, exercise, and creative activities such as art can help the brain mature and learn.

Many Mental Disorders May Begin to Appear during Adolescence

Ongoing changes in the brain, along with physical, emotional, and social changes, can make teens vulnerable to mental-health problems. All the big changes the brain is experiencing may explain why adolescence is a time when many mental disorders—such as schizophrenia, anxiety, depression, bipolar disorder, and eating disorders—can emerge.

Teen Brains May Be More Vulnerable to Stress

Because the teen brain is still developing, teens may respond to stress differently than adults, which could lead to stress-related mental disorders such as anxiety and depression. Mindfulness, which is a psychological process of actively paying attention to the present moment, may help teens cope with and reduce stress.

Teens Need More Sleep than Children and Adults

Research shows that melatonin (the "sleep hormone") levels in the blood are naturally higher later at night and drop later in the morning in teens than in most children and adults. This difference may explain why many teens stay up late and struggle with getting up in the morning. Teens should get about 9 to 10 hours of sleep a night, but most teens do not get enough sleep. A lack of sleep can make it difficult to pay attention, may increase impulsivity, and may increase the risk for irritability or depression.

The Teen Brain Is Resilient

Although adolescence is a vulnerable time for the brain and for teenagers in general, most teens go on to become healthy adults. Some changes in the brain during this important phase of development actually may help protect against long-term mental disorders.

CHAPTER 3
BRAIN CIRCUITS INVOLVED IN MENTAL DISORDERS

About This Chapter: This chapter includes text excerpted from "Brain Basics," National Institute of Mental Health (NIMH), July 27, 2011. Reviewed August 2020.

Mental disorders are common. You may have a friend, colleague, or relative with a mental disorder, or perhaps you have experienced one yourself at some point. Such disorders include depression, anxiety disorders, bipolar disorder, attention deficit hyperactivity disorder (ADHD), and many others.

Some people who develop a mental illness may recover completely; others may have repeated episodes of illness with relatively stable periods in between. Still, others live with symptoms of mental illness every day. They can be moderate or serious, and cause severe disability.

Through research, it is known that mental disorders are brain disorders. Evidence shows that they can be related to changes in the anatomy, physiology, and chemistry of the nervous system. When the brain cannot effectively coordinate the billions of cells in the body, the results can affect many aspects of life. Scientists are continually learning more about how the brain grows and works in healthy people, and how normal brain development and function can go awry, leading to mental illnesses.

Inside the Brain: Neurons and Neural Circuits

Neurons are the basic working unit of the brain and nervous system. These cells are highly specialized for the function of conducting messages. A neuron has three basic parts:

- **Cell body,** which includes the nucleus, cytoplasm, and cell organelles. The nucleus contains DNA and information that the cell needs for growth, metabolism, and repair. Cytoplasm is the substance that fills a cell, including all the chemicals and parts needed for the cell to work properly including small structures called "cell organelles."

- **Dendrites** branch off from the cell body and act as a neuron's point of contact for receiving chemical and electrical signals called "impulses" from neighboring neurons.
- **Axon,** which sends impulses and extends from cell bodies to meet and deliver impulses to another nerve cell. Axons can range in length from a fraction of an inch to several feet.

Each neuron is enclosed by a cell membrane, which separates the inside contents of the cell from its surrounding environment and controls what enters and leaves the cell, and responds to signals from the environment; this all helps the cell maintain its balance with the environment.

Synapses are tiny gaps between neurons, where messages move from one neuron to another as chemical or electrical signals.

The brain begins as a small group of cells in the outer layer of a developing embryo. As the cells grow and differentiate, neurons travel from a central "birthplace" to their final destination. Chemical signals from other cells guide neurons in forming various brain structures. Neighbouring neurons make connections with each other and with distant nerve cells (via axons) to form brain circuits. These circuits control specific body functions such as sleep and speech. The brain continues maturing well into a person's early 20s. Knowing how the brain is wired and how the normal brain's structure develops and matures helps scientists understand what goes wrong in mental illnesses.

Scientists have already begun to chart how the brain develops over time in healthy people and are working to compare that with brain development in people with mental disorders. Genes and environmental cues both help to direct this growth.

Neurotransmitters

Everything we do relies on neurons communicating with one another. Electrical impulses and chemical signals carry messages across different parts of the brain and between the brain and the rest of the nervous system.

When a neuron is activated a small difference in electrical charge occurs. This unbalanced charge is called an "action potential" and is caused by the concentration of ions (atoms or molecules with unbalanced charges) across the cell membrane. The action potential travels very quickly along the axon, like when a line of dominoes falls.

When the action potential reaches the end of an axon, most neurons release a chemical message (a neurotransmitter) which crosses the synapse and binds to receptors on the receiving neuron's dendrites and starts the process over again. At the end of the line, a neurotransmitter may stimulate a different kind of cell (like a gland cell), or may trigger a new chain of messages.

Neurotransmitters send chemical messages between neurons. Mental illnesses, such as depression, can occur when this process does not work correctly.

Communication between neurons can also be electrical, such as in areas of the brain that control movement. When electrical signals are abnormal, they can cause tremors or symptoms found in Parkinson disease (PD).

Brain Regions

Just as many neurons working together form a circuit, many circuits working together form specialized brain systems. We have many specialized brain systems that work across specific brain regions to help us talk, help us make sense of what we see, and help us to solve a problem. Some of the regions most commonly studied in mental-health research are listed below.

- **Amygdala.** The brain's "fear hub," which activates our natural "fight-or-flight" response to confront or escape from a dangerous situation. The amygdala also appears to be involved in learning to fear an event, such as touching a hot stove, and learning not to fear, such as overcoming a fear of spiders. Studying how the amygdala helps create memories of fear and safety may help improve treatments for anxiety disorders like phobias or posttraumatic stress disorder (PTSD).
- **Prefrontal cortex (PFC).** Seat of the brain's executive functions, such as judgement, decision making, and problem-solving. Different parts of the PFC are involved in using short-term or "working" memory and in retrieving long-term memories. This area of the brain also helps to control the amygdala during stressful events. Some research shows that people who have PTSD or ADHD have reduced activity in their PFCs.
- **Anterior cingulate cortex (ACC).** The ACC has many different roles, from controlling blood pressure and heart rate to responding when we sense a mistake, helping us feel motivated and stay focused on a task, and managing proper emotional reactions. Reduced ACC activity or damage to this brain area has been linked to disorders such as ADHD, schizophrenia, and depression.
- **Hippocampus.** Helps create and file new memories. When the hippocampus is damaged, a person cannot create new memories, but can still remember past events and learned skills, and carry on a conversation, all which rely on different parts of the brain. The hippocampus may be involved in mood disorders through its control of a major mood circuit called the "hypothalamic-pituitary-adrenal" (HPA) axis.

CHAPTER 4
COMMON MENTAL DISORDERS IN YOUNG ADULTS

About This Chapter: This chapter includes text excerpted from "Common Mental Health Disorders in Adolescence," Office of Adolescent Health (OAH), U.S. Department of Health and Human Services (HHS), May 1, 2019.

Common mental-health disorders in adolescence include those related to anxiety, depression, attention deficit hyperactivity, and eating.

Anxiety Disorders
- Characterized by feelings of excessive uneasiness, worry, and fear
- Occur in approximately 32 percent of 13- to 18-year-olds
- Examples include generalized anxiety disorder (GAD), posttraumatic stress disorder (PTSD), social anxiety disorder (SAD), obsessive-compulsive disorder (OCD), and phobias

Depression
- Depressed mood that affects thoughts, feelings, and daily activities, including eating, sleeping, and working
- Occurs in approximately 13 percent of 12- to 17-year-olds
- Examples include depressive disorder, postpartum depression, and SAD

Did You Know?
The number of adolescents ages 12 to 17 who experienced a major depressive episode was higher in 2016 than in any year in the previous decade.

Attention Deficit Hyperactivity Disorder

- Characterized by continued inattention and/or hyperactivity-impulsivity that interferes with daily functioning or development
- Occurs in approximately nine percent of 13- to 18-year-olds

Eating Disorders

- Characterized by extreme and abnormal eating behaviors, such as insufficient or excessive eating
- Occur in almost three percent of 13- to 18-year-olds
- Examples include anorexia nervosa, bulimia, and binge eating disorder (BED)

Co-Occurring Disorders

When a person has a mental-health and substance-use disorder at the same time, they have co-occurring disorders. Compared to the general population, people with mental-health disorders are more likely to experience a substance use disorder, repeatedly use alcohol and/or drugs to the point of impairment, and neglect major responsibilities at home, work, or school. Youth who have experienced a major depressive episode are twice as likely to start using alcohol or an illicit drug. A 2010 study found that more than 29 percent of youth who started using alcohol within the past year did so after a major depressive episode, compared to 14.5 percent of youth who had not experienced a major depressive episode. The same pattern also occurred with the use of illicit drugs.

Substance use shares many characteristics with mental illness. Prevention efforts and early treatment are beneficial for people who are at risk for both substance-use and mental-health disorders. A recent U.S. Surgeon General's report (addiction.surgeon general.gov) highlights the scope of substance use (including alcohol) and its negative health impacts for individuals and the nation. Because mental-health and substance use disorders are complicated and involve biological, psychological, and social elements, the Substance Abuse and Mental Health Services Administration (SAMHSA) supports an integrated treatment approach to co-occurring disorders. This approach allows practitioners to comprehensively address symptoms and underlying causes, which often lowers the cost of treatment and leads to better outcomes.

Substance use is not the only disorder that occurs at the same time as mental-health disorders. Different mental-health disorders can occur together (such as anxiety and depression) or mental-health disorders can overlap with physical health disorders (such as depression and diabetes). Symptoms of mental-health disorders can also be similar to other conditions. For example, autism spectrum disorder (ASD) is the name for a group of developmental disorders often characterized by impairments in the ability to communicate and interact with others. ASD includes a wide range of symptoms, skills, and levels of disability. These disorders occur in about

1.5 percent of children and often co-occur with disorders such as depression, anxiety, and sensory integration disorder.

Current Research

Much of the current research on mental health is focused on addressing three areas: the role of trauma and toxic stress in the development of mental-health disorders; factors that promote resilience in the face of challenges; and interventions that include therapeutic or preventive approaches, such as mindfulness meditation.

The federally-funded Adolescent Brain Cognitive Development (ABCD) study was launched in 2016, and will follow the biological and behavioral development of more than 10,000 children from ages 9 to 10 through adolescence and into early adulthood. Researchers will use advanced brain imaging, interviews, and behavioral testing to examine how childhood experiences affect a child's changing biology and vice versa. The interaction between childhood activities and biology could affect brain development and—ultimately—social, behavioral, academic, health, and other outcomes.

Other researchers are interested in understanding the role of medication treating mental-health disorders. Most children who receive outpatient care for mental health see their primary care provider, rather than a specialist, such as a psychiatrist. Primary care providers are more likely than specialists to prescribe medication. Treating a mental-health disorder with medication sometimes requires going through several trials before settling on the most effective medication or combination of medications for the individual. Identifying the best treatment can be stressful and expensive for families. Because of the importance of identifying the best treatments early, the National Institute of Mental Health (NIMH) Mental Health Services Research Committee (SERV) is funding evaluations of the effectiveness of mental-health services and treatments, the use of medication to treat mental-health disorders, service needs for specific populations or for those with co-occurring disorders, and innovative service delivery models.

CHAPTER 5
MENTAL HEALTH: MYTHS AND FACTS

About This Chapter: This chapter includes text excerpted from "Mental Health Myths and Facts," MentalHealth.gov, U.S. Department of Health and Human Services (HHS), August 29, 2017.

Can you tell the difference between a mental-health myth and fact? Learn the truth about the most common mental-health myths.

Mental-Health Problems Affect Everyone

Myth: Mental-health problems do not affect me.

Fact: Mental-health problems are actually very common. In 2014, about:

- One in five American adults experienced a mental-health issue
- One in 10 young people experienced a period of major depression
- One in 25 Americans lived with a serious mental illness, such as schizophrenia, bipolar disorder, or major depression

Suicide is the 10th leading cause of death in the United States. It accounts for the loss of more than 41,000 American lives each year, more than double the number of lives lost to homicide.

Myth: Children do not experience mental-health problems.

Fact: Even very young children may show early warning signs of mental-health concerns. These mental-health problems are often clinically diagnosable, and can be a product of the interaction of biological, psychological, and social factors.

Half of all mental-health disorders show first signs before a person turns 14 years old, and three-quarters of mental-health disorders begin before age 24.

Unfortunately, less than 20 percent of children and adolescents with diagnosable mental-health problems receive the treatment they need. Early mental-health support can help a child before problems interfere with other developmental needs.

Myth: People with mental-health problems are violent and unpredictable.

Fact: The vast majority of people with mental-health problems are no more likely to be violent than anyone else. Most people with mental illness are not violent and only 3 percent to 5 percent of violent acts can be attributed to individuals living with a serious mental illness. In fact, people with severe mental illnesses are over 10 times more likely to be victims of violent crime than the general population. You probably know someone with a mental-health problem and do not even realize it, because many people with mental-health problems are highly active and productive members of our communities.

Myth: People with mental-health needs, even those who are managing their mental illness, cannot tolerate the stress of holding down a job.

Fact: People with mental-health problems are just as productive as other employees. Employers who hire people with mental-health problems report good attendance and punctuality as well as motivation, good work, and job tenure on par with or greater than other employees.

When employees with mental-health problems receive effective treatment, it can result in:

- Lower total medical costs
- Increased productivity
- Lower absenteeism
- Decreased disability costs

Myth: Personality weakness or character flaws cause mental-health problems. People with mental-health problems can snap out of it if they try hard enough.

Fact: Mental-health problems have nothing to do with being lazy or weak and many people need help to get better. Many factors contribute to mental-health problems, including:

- Biological factors such as genes, physical illness, injury, or brain chemistry
- Life experiences, such as trauma or a history of abuse
- Family history of mental-health problems

People with mental-health problems can get better and many recover completely.

Helping Individuals with Mental-Health Problems

Myth: There is no hope for people with mental-health problems. Once a friend or family member develops mental-health problems, she or he will never recover.

Fact: Studies show that people with mental-health problems get better and many recover completely. "Recovery" refers to the process in which people are able to live, work, learn, and participate fully in their communities. There are more treatments, services, and community support systems than ever before, and they work.

Myth: Therapy and self-help are a waste of time. Why bother when you can just take a pill?

Fact: Treatment for mental-health problems varies depending on the individual and could include medication, therapy, or both. Many individuals work with a support system during the healing and recovery process.

Myth: I cannot do anything for a person with a mental-health problem.

Fact: Friends and loved ones can make a big difference. Only 44 percent of adults with diagnosable mental-health problems and less than 20 percent of children and adolescents receive needed treatment. Friends and family can be important influences to help someone get the treatment and services they need by:

- Reaching out and letting them know you are available to help
- Helping them access mental-health services
- Learning and sharing the facts about mental health, especially if you hear something that is not true
- Treating them with respect, just as you would anyone else
- Refusing to define them by their diagnosis or using labels such as "crazy"

Myth: Prevention does not work. It is impossible to prevent mental illnesses.

Fact: Prevention of mental, emotional, and behavioral disorders focuses on addressing known risk factors such as exposure to trauma that can affect the chances that children, youth, and young adults will develop mental-health problems. Promoting the social-emotional well-being of children and youth leads to:

- Higher overall productivity
- Better educational outcomes
- Lower crime rates
- Stronger economies
- Lower healthcare costs
- Improved quality of life
- Increased lifespan
- Improved family life

CHAPTER 6

ANXIETY DISORDERS: WHEN PANIC, FEAR, AND WORRIES OVERWHELM

About This Chapter: This chapter includes text excerpted from "Understanding Anxiety Disorders," *NIH News in Health*, National Institutes of Health (NIH), March 2016. Reviewed August 2020.

Many of us worry from time to time. You fret over finances, feel anxious about job interviews, or get nervous about social gatherings. These feelings can be normal or even helpful. They may give us a boost of energy or help us focus. But, for people with anxiety disorders, they can be overwhelming.

Anxiety disorders affect nearly 1 in 5 American adults each year. People with these disorders have feelings of fear and uncertainty that interfere with everyday activities and last for six months or more. Anxiety disorders can also raise your risk for other medical problems such as heart disease, diabetes, substance abuse, and depression.

The good news is that most anxiety disorders get better with therapy. The course of treatment depends on the type of anxiety disorder. Medications, psychotherapy ("talk therapy"), or a combination of both can usually relieve troubling symptoms.

"Anxiety disorders are one of the most treatable mental-health problems we see," says Dr. Daniel Pine, a National Institutes of Health (NIH) neuroscientist and psychiatrist. "Still, for reasons we do not fully understand, most people who have these problems do not get the treatments that could really help them."

One of the most common types of anxiety disorder is social anxiety disorder (SAD), or social phobia. It affects both women and men equally—a total of about 15 million United States adults. Without treatment, social phobia can last for years or even a lifetime. People with social phobia may worry for days or weeks before a social event. They are often embarrassed, self-conscious, and afraid of being judged. They find it hard to talk to others. They may blush, sweat, tremble, or feel sick to their stomach when around other people.

Other common types of anxiety disorders include generalized anxiety disorder (GAD), which affects nearly 7 million American adults, and panic disorder, which affects about 6 million. Both are twice as common in women as in men.

People with GAD worry endlessly over everyday issues—like health, money, or family problems—even if they realize there is little cause for concern. They startle easily, cannot relax, and cannot concentrate. They find it hard to fall asleep or stay asleep. They may get headaches, muscle aches, or unexplained pains. Symptoms often get worse during times of stress.

People with panic disorder have sudden, repeated bouts of fear—called "panic attacks"—that last several minutes or more. During a panic attack, they may feel that they cannot breathe or that they are having a heart attack. They may fear loss of control or feel a sense of unreality. Not everyone who has panic attacks will develop panic disorder. But, if the attacks recur without warning, creating fear of having another attack at any time, then it is likely panic disorder.

Anxiety disorders tend to run in families. But, researchers are not certain why some family members develop these conditions while others do not. No specific genes have been found to actually cause an anxiety disorder. "Many different factors—including genes, stress, and the environment—have small effects that add up in complex ways to affect a person's risk for these disorders," Pine says.

"Many kids with anxiety disorders will outgrow their conditions. But, most anxiety problems you see in adults started during their childhood," Pine adds.

"Anxiety disorders are among the most common psychiatric disorders in children, with an estimated 1 in 3 suffering anxiety at some point during childhood or adolescence," says Dr. Susan Whitfield-Gabrieli, a brain imaging expert at the Massachusetts Institute of Technology (MIT). "About half of diagnosable mental-health disorders start by age 14, so there is a lot of interest in uncovering the factors that might influence the brain by those early teen years."

Whitfield-Gabrieli is launching an NIH-funded study to create detailed magnetic resonance imaging (MRI) images of the brains of more than 200 teens, ages 14 to 15, with and without anxiety or depression. The scientists will then assess what brain structures and activities might be linked to these conditions. The study is part of the NIH's Human Connectome Project (HCP), in which research teams across the country are studying the complex brain connections that affect health and disease.

Whitfield-Gabrieli and colleagues have shown that analysis of brain connections might help predict which adults with social phobia will likely respond to cognitive-behavioral therapy (CBT). CBT is a type of talk therapy known to be effective for people with anxiety disorders. It helps them change their thinking patterns and how they react to anxiety-provoking situations. But, it does not work for everyone.

Of 38 adults with social phobia, those who responded best after 3 months of CBT had similar patterns of brain connections. This brain analysis led to major improvement, compared to a clinician's assessment alone, in predicting treatment response. Larger studies will be needed to confirm the benefits of the approach.

Troubled by Anxiety?

If feelings of anxiety seem overwhelming or interfere with every-day activities:

- See your family doctor or nurse practitioner.
- The next step may be talking to a mental-health professional. Consider finding someone trained in CBT who is also open to using medication if needed. You may need to try several medicines before finding the right one.
- Consider joining a self-help or support group to share problems and achievements with others.
- Stress management techniques and mindfulness meditation may help relieve anxiety symptoms.

"Ultimately, we hope that brain imaging will help us predict clinical outcomes and actually tailor the treatment to each individual—to know whether they will respond best to psychotherapy or to certain medications," Whitfield-Gabrieli says.

Other researchers are focusing on our emotions and our ability to adjust them. "We want to understand not only how emotions can help us, but also how they can create difficulties if they are of the wrong intensity or the wrong type for a particular situation," says Dr. James Gross, a clinical psychologist at Stanford University.

We all use different strategies to adjust our emotions, often without thinking about it. If something makes you angry, you may try to tamp down your emotion to avoid making a scene. If something annoys you, you might try to ignore it, modify it, or entirely avoid it.

But, these strategies can turn harmful over time. For instance, people with social phobia might decide to avoid attending a professional conference so they can keep their anxiety in check. That makes them lose opportunities at work and miss chances to meet people and make friends.

Gross and others are examining the differences between how people with and without anxiety disorders regulate their emotions. "We are finding that CBT is helpful in part because it teaches people to more effectively use emotion regulation strategies," Gross says. "They then become more competent in their ability to use these strategies in their everyday lives."

"It is important to be aware that many different kinds of treatments are available, and people with anxiety disorders tend to have very good responses to those treatments," Pine adds. The best way to start is often by talking with your physician. If you are a parent, talk with your child's pediatrician. "These health professionals are generally prepared to help identify such problems and help patients get the appropriate care they need," Pine says.

CHAPTER 7
DEPRESSION IN TEENS: GET THE FACTS

About This Chapter: This chapter includes text excerpted from "Teen Depression," National Institute of Mental Health (NIMH), April 26, 2011. Reviewed August 2020.

Being a teenager can be tough. There are changes taking place in your body and brain that can affect how you learn, think, and behave. And if you are facing tough or stressful situations, it is normal to have emotional ups and downs.

But if you have been overwhelmingly sad for a long time (a few weeks to months) and you are not able to concentrate or do the things you usually enjoy, you may want to talk to a trusted adult about depression.

What Is Depression?
Depression (major depressive disorder) is a medical illness that can interfere with your ability to handle your daily activities, such as sleeping, eating, or managing your schoolwork. Depression is common but that does not mean it is not serious. Treatment may be needed for someone to feel better. Depression can happen at any age, but often symptoms begin in the teens or early 20s or 30s. It can occur along with other mental disorders, substance abuse, and other health conditions.

Why Can You Not Just 'Snap Out' of Depression?
Well-meaning friends or family members may try to tell someone with depression to "snap out of it," "just be positive," or "you can be happier if you just try harder." But depression is not a sign of weakness or a character flaw. Most people with depression need treatment to get better.

What Are the Signs and Symptoms of Depression?
Sadness is something we all experience. It is a normal reaction to a loss or a setback, but it usually passes with a little time. Depression is different.

If you are wondering if you may have depression, ask yourself these questions:
- Do you constantly feel sad, anxious, or even "empty," like you feel nothing?

- Do you feel hopeless or like everything is going wrong?
- Do you feel like you are worthless or helpless? Do you feel guilty about things?
- Do you feel irritable much of the time?
- Do you find yourself spending more time alone and withdrawing from friends and family?
- Are your grades dropping?
- Have you lost interest or pleasure in activities and hobbies that you used to enjoy?
- Have your eating or sleeping habits changed (eating or sleeping more than usual or less than usual)?
- Do you always feel tired? Like you have less energy than normal or no energy at all?
- Do you feel restless or have trouble sitting still?
- Do you feel like you have trouble concentrating, remembering information, or making decisions?
- Do you have aches or pains, headaches, cramps, or stomach problems without a clear cause?
- Do you ever think about dying or suicide? Have you ever tried to harm yourself?

Not everyone with depression experiences every symptom. Some people experience only a few symptoms. Others may have many. The symptoms and how long they last will vary from person to person.

How Do You Get Help?

If you think you might have depression, you are not alone. Depression is common, but it is also treatable. Ask for help! Here are a few steps you can take:

- **Step 1.** Try talking to a trusted adult, such as your parent or guardian, your teacher, or a school counselor. If you do not feel comfortable speaking to an adult, try talking to a friend. If you are not sure where to turn, you can use TXT 4 HELP Interactive (www.nationalsafeplace.org/txt-4-help), which allows you to text live with a mental-health professional. For more ideas and a list of health hotlines, visit www.nimh.nih.gov (search words: children and adolescents).
- **Step 2.** If you are under the age of 18, ask your parent or guardian to make an appointment with your doctor for an evaluation. Your doctor can make sure you do not have a physical illness that may be affecting your mental health. Your doctor may also talk to you about the possibility of seeing a mental-health professional, such as a psychiatrist, counselor, psychologist, or therapist. These practitioners can diagnose and treat depression and other mental disorders.

Although antidepressants can be effective, they may present serious risks to some, especially children and teens. Anyone taking antidepressants should be monitored closely, especially when they first start taking them. Severe anxiety or agitation early in treatment can be especially distressing and should be reported to the doctor immediately.

For many people, the risks of untreated depression outweigh the side effects of antidepressant medications when they are used under a doctor's careful supervision. Information about medications changes frequently. Talk to your doctor and visit the U.S. Food and Drug Administration (FDA) website (www.fda.gov) for the latest safety information.

How Is Depression Treated?

Depression is usually treated with psychotherapy, medication, or a combination of the two.

What Is Psychotherapy?

Psychotherapy (sometimes called "talk therapy") is a term for treatment techniques that can help you identify and manage troubling emotions, thoughts, and behavior. Psychotherapy can take place in a one-on-one meeting with you and a licensed mental-health professional. Sometimes you might be part of a group guided by a mental-health professional.

What Medications Treat Depression

If your doctor thinks you need medicine to treat your depression, she or he might prescribe an antidepressant.

When you are taking an antidepressant, it is important to carefully follow your doctor's directions for taking your medicine. The medication could take up to six weeks to work and you should not stop taking it without the help of a doctor. You should also avoid using alcohol or drugs that have not been prescribed to you so that your medications can work.

When it is time to stop the medication, the doctor will help you slowly and safely decrease the dose so that your body can adjust. If you stop taking the medication too soon, your depression symptoms may return. Another reason to stop medication gradually is that stopping suddenly can cause withdrawal symptoms like anxiety and irritability.

Antidepressants can have side effects. These side effects are usually mild (possible stomach upsets or headaches) and may go away on their own. But talk to your doctor about any side effects that you experience because your doctor might adjust the dose or change the medicine.

What Else Can You Do to Help Manage Your Depression?

Be patient and know that treatment takes time to work. In the meantime, you can:

- Stay active and exercise, even if it is just going for a walk.
- Try to keep a regular sleep schedule.
- Spend time with friends and family.
- Break down school or work tasks into smaller ones and organize them in order of what needs to get done first. Then, do what you can.

What Can You Do If Someone You Know Might Have Depression?

If you think your friend might have depression, first help her or him talk to a trusted adult who can connect your friend to a health professional. You can also:
- Be supportive, patient, and encouraging, even if you do not fully understand what is going on.
- Invite your friend to activities, social events, or just to hang out.
- Remind your friend that getting help is important and that with time and treatment, she or he will feel better.

Never ignore comments about death and suicide, even if it seems like a joke or overdramatic. Talking about suicide is not just a bid for attention but should be taken seriously. Talk to a trusted adult such as a parent, teacher, or older sibling as soon as you can.

What Should You Do If Someone You Know Is Considering Suicide?

Often, family and friends are the first to recognize the warning signs of suicide and can take the first step toward helping the person find help.

Remember:
- If someone is telling you that she or he is going to kill herself or himself, do not leave her or him alone.
- Do not promise anyone that you will keep her or his suicidal thoughts a secret. Make sure to tell a trusted friend or family member, or an adult with whom you feel comfortable.
- Get help as soon as possible. Call 911 for emergency services and/or take the person to the nearest hospital emergency room.

You can also call 800-273-TALK (800-273-8255), the toll-free number for the National Suicide Prevention Lifeline, which is available 24 hours a day, every day. The service is available to everyone. All calls are free and confidential. You can also chat with the NSPL online (www.suicidepreventionlifeline.org).

The Crisis Text Line (www.crisistextline.org) is another free, confidential resource available 24 hours a day, seven days a week. Text "HOME" to 741741 and a trained crisis counselor will respond to you with support and information via text message.

What If Someone Is Posting Suicidal Messages or Something Disturbing on Social Media?

If you see messages or live streaming suicidal behavior on social media, call 911 immediately, contact the toll-free National Suicide Prevention Lifeline at 800-273-TALK (800-273-8255), or text the Crisis Text Line (text HOME to 741741).

Some social media sites also have a process to report suicidal content and get help for the person posting the message. Each offers different options on how to respond if you see concerning posts about suicide. For example:

- Facebook Suicide Prevention webpage can be found at www.facebook.com/help/594991777257121 [use the search term "suicide" or "suicide prevention"].
- Instagram uses automated tools in the app to provide resources, which can also be found online at help.instagram.com [use the search term, "suicide," "self-injury," or "suicide prevention"].
- Snapchat's Support provides guidance at support.snapchat.com [use the search term, "suicide" or "suicide prevention"].
- Tumblr Counseling and Prevention Resources webpage can be found at tumblr.zendesk.com [use the search term "counseling" or "prevention," then click on "Counseling and prevention resources"].
- Twitter's Best Practices in Dealing With Self-Harm and Suicide at support.twitter.com [use the search term "suicide," "self-harm," or "suicide prevention"].
- YouTube's Safety Center webpage can be found at support.google.com/youtube [use the search term "suicide and self-injury"].

Because help via these processes may be delayed, it is still important to call 911 if someone is posting suicidal messages or something disturbing on social media. People—even strangers—have saved lives by being vigilant.

CHAPTER 8
RISK AND PROTECTIVE FACTORS

About This Chapter: This chapter includes text excerpted from "Mental Health—Risk and Protective Factors," Youth.gov, April 10, 2018.

As youth grow and reach their developmental competencies, there are contextual variables that promote or hinder the process. These are frequently referred to as "protective and risk factors."

The presence or absence and various combinations of protective and risk factors contribute to the mental health of youth. Identifying protective and risk factors in youth may guide the prevention and intervention strategies to pursue with them. Protective and risk factors may also influence the course mental-health disorders might take if present.

A protective factor can be defined as "a characteristic at the biological, psychological, family, or community (including peers and culture) level that is associated with a lower likelihood of problem outcomes or that reduces the negative impact of a risk factor on problem outcomes." Conversely, a risk factor can be defined as "a characteristic at the biological, psychological, family, community, or cultural level that precedes and is associated with a higher likelihood of problem outcomes." Table 8.1 provides examples of protective and risk factors by five domains: youth, family, peer, community, and society.

Risk and Protective Factors for Mental, Emotional, and Behavioral Disorders in Adolescents

Table 8.1. Examples of Protective and Risk Factors by Five Domains: Youth, Family, Peer, Community, and Society

Risk Factors	Domains	Protective Factors
• Female gender • Early puberty • Difficult temperament: inflexibility, low positive mood, withdrawal, poor concentration • Low self-esteem, perceived incompetence, negative explanatory and inferential style • Anxiety • Low-level depressive symptoms and dysthymia • Insecure attachment • Poor social skills: communication and problem-solving skills • Extreme need for approval and social support • Low self-esteem • Shyness • Emotional problems in childhood • Conduct disorder • Favorable attitudes toward drugs • Rebelliousness • Early substance use • Antisocial behavior • Head injury • Marijuana use • Childhood exposure to lead or mercury (neurotoxins)	Individual	• Positive physical development • Academic achievement/intellectual development • High self-esteem • Emotional self-regulation • Good coping skills and problem-solving skills • Engagement and connections in two or more of the following contexts: school, with peers, in athletics, employment, religion, culture
• Parental depression • Parent-child conflict • Poor parenting • Negative family environment (may include substance abuse in parents) • Child abuse/maltreatment • Single-parent family (for girls only) • Divorce • Marital conflict • Family conflict	Family	• Family provides structure, limits, rules, monitoring, and predictability • Supportive relationships with family members • Clear expectations for behavior and values

Table 8.1. Continued

Risk Factors	Domains	Protective Factors
• Parent with anxiety • Parental/marital conflict • Family conflict (interactions between parents and children and among children) • Parental drug/alcohol use • Parental unemployment • Substance use among parents • Lack of adult supervision • Poor attachment with parents • Family dysfunction • Family member with schizophrenia • Poor parental supervision • Parental depression • Sexual abuse		
• Peer rejection • Stressful events • Poor academic achievement • Poverty • Community-level stressful or traumatic events • School-level stressful or traumatic events • Community violence • School violence • Poverty • Traumatic event • School failure • Low commitment to school • Not college bound • Aggression toward peers • Associating with drug-using peers • Societal/community norms favor alcohol and drug use • Urban setting • Poverty • Associating with deviant peers • Loss of close relationship or friends	School, neighborhood, and community	• Presence of mentors and support for development of skills and interests • Opportunities for engagement within school and community • Positive norms • Clear expectations for behavior • Physical and psychological safety

CHAPTER 9
IMPORTANCE OF MENTAL-HEALTH PROMOTION AND PREVENTION

About This Chapter: This chapter includes text excerpted from "Mental Health—Promotion and Prevention," Youth.gov, February 5, 2017.

The term "mental-health promotion and prevention" have often been confused. "Promotion" is defined as intervening to optimize positive mental health by addressing determinants of positive mental health before a specific mental-health problem has been identified, with the ultimate goal of improving the positive mental health of the population. "Mental-health prevention" is defined as intervening to minimize mental-health problems by addressing determinants of mental-health problems before a specific mental-health problem has been identified in the individual, group, or population of focus with the ultimate goal of reducing the number of future mental-health problems in the population. Mental-health promotion and prevention are at the core of a public-health approach to children and youth mental health which addresses the mental health of all children, focusing on the balance of optimizing positive mental health as well as preventing and treating mental-health problems.

Promotion

Mental-health promotion attempts to encourage and increase protective factors and healthy behaviors that can help prevent the onset of a diagnosable mental disorder and reduce risk factors that can lead to the development of a mental disorder. It also involves creating living conditions and environments that support mental health and allow people to adopt and maintain healthy lifestyles or a climate that respects and protects basic civil, political, socioeconomic, and cultural rights is fundamental to mental-health promotion. Without the security and freedom provided by these rights, it is very difficult to maintain a high level of mental health."

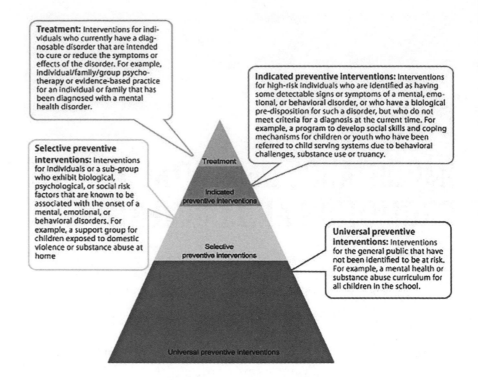

Treatment: Interventions for individuals who currently have a diagnosable disorder that are intended to cure or reduce the symptoms or effects of the disorder. For example, individual/family/group psychotherapy or evidence-based practice for an individual or family that has been diagnosed with a mental health disorder.

Selective preventive interventions: Interventions for individuals or a sub-group who exhibit biological, psychological, or social risk factors that are known to be associated with the onset of a mental, emotional, or behavioral disorders. For example, a support group for children exposed to domestic violence or substance abuse at home

Indicated preventive interventions: Interventions for high-risk individuals who are identified as having some detectable signs or symptoms of a mental, emotional, or behavioral disorder, or who have a biological pre-disposition for such a disorder, but who do not meet criteria for a diagnosis at the current time. For example, a program to develop social skills and coping mechanisms for children or youth who have been referred to child serving systems due to behavioral challenges, substance use or truancy.

Universal preventive interventions: Interventions for the general public that have not been identified to be at risk. For example, a mental health or substance abuse curriculum for all children in the school.

Treatment

Indicated preventive interventions

Selective preventive interventions

Universal preventive interventions

Figure 9.1. Levels of Intervention

Specifically, mental health can be promoted through:
- Early childhood interventions (e.g., home visits for pregnant women, preschool psychosocial activities)
- Providing support for children (e.g., skill-building programs, child and youth development programs)
- Programs targeted at vulnerable groups, including minorities, indigenous people, migrants, and people affected by conflicts and disasters (e.g., psychosocial interventions after disasters)
- Incorporating mental-health promotional activities in schools (e.g., programs supporting ecological changes in schools and child-friendly schools)
- Violence prevention programs and among others
- Community development programs

"Positive youth development" is defined by the Interagency Working Group on Youth Programs (IWGYP) as an intentional, prosocial approach that:
- Engages youth within their communities, schools, organizations, peer groups, and families in a manner that is productive and constructive

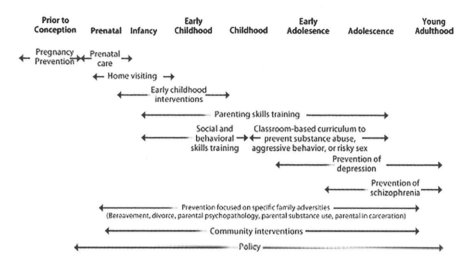

Interventions by Developmental Phase

Figure 9.2. Preventive Interventions by Developmental Phase

- Recognizes, utilizes, and enhances youths' strengths and promotes positive outcomes for young people by providing opportunities, fostering positive relationships
- Furnishing the support needed to build on their leadership strengths

It provides a lens for promoting the mental health of youth by focusing on protective factors in a young person's environment, and on how these factors could influence one's ability to overcome adversity.

Prevention

Prevention efforts can vary based on the audience they are addressing, level of intensity they are providing, and the development phase they target. Figure 9.1 depicts the different types of prevention as defined by the Institute of Medicine (IOM). As prevention efforts move from universal prevention interventions to treatment they increase in intensity and become more individualized.

Interventions may vary not only based on level of intensity, as seen in Figure 9.1, but also on the development phase of the youth. Figure 9.2 provides examples of preventive interventions for each of the developmental stages through young adulthood.

PART 2 | MAJOR TYPES OF ANXIETY DISORDERS AND DEPRESSION

CHAPTER 10
GENERALIZED ANXIETY DISORDER

About This Chapter: This chapter includes text excerpted from "Generalized Anxiety Disorder: When Worry Gets Out of Control," National Institute of Mental Health (NIMH), 2016. Reviewed August 2020.

What Is Generalized Anxiety Disorder?

Occasional anxiety is a normal part of life. You might worry about things like health, money, or family problems. But, people with generalized anxiety disorder (GAD) feel extremely worried or feel nervous about these and other things—even when there is little or no reason to worry about them. People with GAD find it difficult to control their anxiety and stay focused on daily tasks.

The good news is that GAD is treatable. Call your doctor to talk about your symptoms so that you can feel better.

What Are the Signs and Symptoms of Generalized Anxiety Disorder?

Generalized anxiety disorder develops slowly. It often starts during the teen years or young adulthood. People with GAD may:

- Worry very much about everyday things
- Have trouble controlling their worries or feelings of nervousness

Prevalence

Approximately 5.7 percent of people will have a diagnosis of GAD at some point in their lifetime, and it is about twice as common in females. Subclinical GAD is even more common than GAD. This is defined as having some symptoms of the disorder, but not enough for a diagnosis to be made. An additional 8 to 13.7 percent of people will experience subclinical GAD at some point in their life. Even though they do not have all the symptoms needed for a diagnosis of GAD, they too have higher levels of distress and impairment in their lives as compared to those without these anxiety symptoms. They are also at risk for developing another psychiatric disorder; between 42 to 86.3 percent of those with subclinical GAD have symptoms or a diagnosis of another disorder.

(Source: "What Is Generalized Anxiety Disorder?" Mental Illness Research, Education and Clinical Center (MIRECC), U.S. Department of Veterans Affairs (VA))

Symptoms may get better or worse at different times, and they are often worse during times of stress, such as with a physical illness, during exams at school, or during a family or relationship conflict.

- Know that they worry much more than they should
- Feel restless and have trouble relaxing
- Have a hard time concentrating
- Be easily startled
- Have trouble falling asleep or staying asleep
- Feel easily tired or tired all the time
- Have headaches, muscle aches, stomach aches, or unexplained pains
- Have a hard time swallowing
- Tremble or twitch
- Be irritable or feel "on edge"
- Sweat a lot, feel light-headed or out of breath
- Have to go to the bathroom a lot

Children and teens with GAD often worry excessively about:
- Their performance, such as in school or in sports
- Catastrophes, such as earthquakes or war

Adults with GAD are often highly nervous about everyday circumstances, such as:
- Job security or performance
- Health
- Finances
- The health and well-being of their children
- Being late
- Completing household chores and other responsibilities

Both children and adults with GAD may experience physical symptoms that make it hard to function and that interfere with daily life.

What Causes Generalized Anxiety Disorder

Generalized anxiety disorder sometimes runs in families, but no one knows for sure why some family members have it while others do not. Researchers have found that several parts of the brain, as well as biological processes, play a key role in fear and anxiety. By learning more about how the brain and body function in people with anxiety disorders, researchers may be able to create better treatments. Researchers are also looking for ways in which stress and environmental factors play a role.

How Is Generalized Anxiety Disorder Treated?

First, talk to your doctor about your symptoms. Your doctor should do an exam and ask you about your health history to make sure that an unrelated physical problem is not causing your symptoms. Your doctor may refer to you a mental-health specialist, such as a psychiatrist or psychologist.

Generalized anxiety disorder is generally treated with psychotherapy, medication, or both. Talk with your doctor about the best treatment for you.

Psychotherapy

A type of psychotherapy called "cognitive-behavioral therapy" (CBT) is especially useful for treating GAD. CBT teaches a person different ways of thinking, behaving, and reacting to situations that help her or him feel less anxious and worried.

Medications

Doctors may also prescribe medication to help treat GAD. Your doctor will work with you to find the best medication and dose for you. Different types of medication can be effective in GAD:

- Selective serotonin reuptake inhibitors (SSRIs)
- Serotonin-norepinephrine reuptake inhibitors (SNRIs)
- Other serotonergic medication
- Benzodiazepines

Doctors commonly use SSRIs and SNRIs to treat depression, but they are also helpful for the symptoms of GAD. They may take several weeks to start working. These medications may also cause side effects, such as headaches, nausea, or difficulty sleeping. These side effects are usually not severe for most people, especially if the dose starts off low and is increased slowly over time. Talk to your doctor about any side effects that you have.

Buspirone is another serotonergic medication that can be helpful in GAD. Buspirone needs to be taken continuously for several weeks for it to be fully effective.

Benzodiazepines, which are sedative medications, can also be used to manage severe forms of GAD. These medications are powerfully effective in rapidly decreasing anxiety, but they can cause tolerance and dependence if you use them continuously. Therefore, your doctor will only prescribe them for brief periods of time if you need them.

Do not give up on treatment too quickly. Both psychotherapy and medication can take some time to work. A healthy lifestyle can also help combat anxiety. Make sure to get enough sleep and exercise, eat a healthy diet, and turn to family and friends who you trust for support.

CHAPTER 11
SEPARATION ANXIETY DISORDER

What Is Separation Anxiety Disorder?

Individuals with separation anxiety disorder (SAD) worry excessively when they anticipate or experience separation from parents or loved ones. Children with SAD experience extreme distress when they are away from parents or caregivers and fear they could get lost from their family or think something bad is happening to their family while they are apart. Separation anxiety is normal in early childhood, but it becomes a disorder when anxiety interferes with age-appropriate activities and behavior. SAD is most often diagnosed in children during preschool and the early school years, but in rare cases, it can become a problem in early adolescence. It is estimated that about 4 percent of all children have this disorder, which can be treated with behavioral and pharmacological therapy if identified early.

What Are the Characteristics of Separation Anxiety Disorder?

Symptoms exhibited with SAD tend to vary with each individual, but some common characteristics include:

- Overattachment to parents or loved ones and a perception of danger to family during separation
- Worry and stress before or during separation from parents or loved ones
- Complaints of headache, nausea, dizziness, or other physical symptoms when separation is anticipated
- Having a hard time saying goodbye to parents, throwing tantrums when faced with separation, feeling afraid of staying alone in one part of a house, or fear of sleeping in a darkened room
- Being afraid of staying home in the absence of parents or loved ones
- Worrisome thoughts of harm to parents or loved ones (e.g., accident, illness, or death)

- Persistent thoughts of the dangers of being separated from loved ones, such as being kidnapped or getting lost
- An overwhelming need to know where parents are when apart, often phoning or texting
- Difficulty falling asleep away from home
- Nightmares with themes of separation from parents or loved ones
- Avoiding playtime, birthday parties, and other activities away from loved ones
- Obsessively shadowing a parent at home or elsewhere
- Refusal to leave home or go to school

What Causes Separation Anxiety Disorder

Biological and environmental factors could all contribute to SAD. Other causes can include chemical imbalances, possibly of such substances as norepinephrine and serotonin in the brain. There could be a biological tendency to feel anxious, but the disorder could also be the result of behavior learned from family members who display elevated anxiety levels around the child. It is also possible that SAD could result from a traumatic childhood experience.

Who Is Affected by Separation Anxiety Disorder?

A certain degree of separation anxiety is normal in children, and dealing with it is a natural part of growing up. SAD is identified when anxiety about being apart from home and family is far beyond that of typical child development. It occurs equally in both sexes, and symptoms usually surface in children following a break from school, such as after Christmas vacation or a period of extended illness. Children of parents with this disorder have a higher than average likelihood of developing the same condition.

How Is Separation Anxiety Disorder Diagnosed?

A child psychiatrist or other mental-health professional diagnoses SAD on the basis of a psychological evaluation. Diagnosis involves identifying and quantifying the distress experienced by the individual during separation from parents or loved ones. Among other factors, the child must experience the symptoms for at least four weeks to meet the technical criteria for SAD. A clinician will be able to determine if the symptoms are otherwise only a temporary response to a stressful life situation.

What Is the Treatment for Separation Anxiety Disorder?

The diagnostician will evaluate the condition of the child and decide on treatment based on the severity of symptoms, age of the child, health and medical history, tolerance for medication and therapy, and personal preference for mode of treatment. The first-line of treatment in SAD is psychotherapy. Cognitive-behavioral therapy (CBT), in particular, has been very successful in mild-to-moderate cases.

The focus of treatment is to provide the child with the skills to manage anxiety and master the situations that contribute to the symptoms of SAD. Exposure therapy, a modified version of CBT is recommended in certain cases. Here, the child is exposed to separation in small, controlled doses, which helps reduce anxiety gradually over time. In severe cases that do not respond to psychotherapy, medication may be required. In such cases, selective serotonin reuptake inhibitors (SSRIs), antidepressants, and antianxiety medications are often prescribed to make the child feel calmer.

How Is Separation Anxiety Disorder Prevented?

Preventive measures are presently unknown. Instead of prevention, the focus is on early detection and intervention, which can successfully reduce the severity of the disorder and enhance normal growth and development patterns, while improving the quality of life for affected children.

References

1. "Separation Anxiety Disorder," Jane and Terry Semel Institute for Neuroscience and Human Behavior, n.d.
2. "Separation Anxiety Disorder," Stanford Children's Health, n.d.
3. "Separation Anxiety Disorder," Child Mind Institute, n.d.

CHAPTER 12
SELECTIVE MUTISM

What Is Selective Mutism?

Selective mutism (SM) is a social anxiety disorder that is most often seen in children that may continue during their teens. Individuals with SM are unable to speak in certain social settings and with certain people. A teen with SM may speak normally with parents and a few others but have difficulty speaking, or speaking above a whisper, in specific settings, such as school, public places, or family gatherings. The condition is quite rare, with few cases documented in school, clinical, and teen-guidance casework.

Teens with SM typically fail to talk in school, which can interfere with academic and social performance. They sometimes communicate nonverbally by nodding, pointing, or writing, but some teens remain motionless and expressionless until others correctly guess what they need. SM can cause considerable distress in certain instances, such as when the teen does not communicate in times of pain or when needing to use the bathroom.

Teens with SM possess the desire to speak but hold back because of anxiety, embarrassment, and shyness. It is important to understand that they do not willfully refuse to speak but rather is unable to do so in particular situations. As a result, they often fail to participate in age-appropriate activities in and outside of school. SM is not to be confused with such behavior as shyness during the first few weeks of school or reticence to speak when a child is adapting to a new language.

What Are the Signs and Symptoms of Selective Mutism?

The diagnostic criteria laid down in the *Diagnostic and Statistical Manual of Mental Disorders, 5th Edition* (DSM-5) include:

- Consistent failure to talk in social situations in which the teen is expected to speak—in school, for example—despite speaking in other situations.

- The inability to talk interferes with educational and occupational achievements or social interaction.
- The problem lasts for at least one month in duration but is not limited to the first month in school.
- The failure to speak in social situations cannot be attributed to lack of knowledge or comfort with using language.
- The condition cannot be explained by communication disorders or mental-health issues, such as autism or schizophrenia.

Teens with SM may also display symptoms related to social anxiety and social phobia, such as:
- Being overly attached to parents
- Being traumatized when asked to respond verbally in public
- Becoming anxious when a picture or video is taken
- Avoiding eating in public
- Being anxious about using public restrooms

Teens with SM avoid conversations in many situations, and if they are able to express themselves, frequently do so by gesturing, nodding, and pointing. They often fear being ignored, ridiculed, or harshly evaluated if they try to speak.

What Are the Causes and Risk Factors of Selective Mutism?

The causes of SM are not yet definitively known, but multiple factors may play a role. For example, some research studies point to genetic influence as a possible cause for a predisposition to the condition. In many cases, it has been found that parents or other family members currently or previously have had symptoms related to extreme shyness, panic attacks, and social anxiety.

Some of the risk factors associated with SM include extreme shyness, a family history of the condition, or an anxiety disorder, such as panic disorder, or obsessive-compulsive behavior. In addition, research has shown that SM is four times more common in immigrant children than in the general population.

How Is Selective Mutism Diagnosed?

Diagnosis of SM is based on the crucial observation that the teen can comprehend language and speak normally but consistently fails to do so in specific settings. For instance, they typically displays appropriate verbal skills at home with parents and certain other individuals with whom they are comfortable. In order to arrive at a diagnosis, a doctor or mental-health professional will rely on reports from parents and other adults who are in contact with the teen to determine patterns across a variety of situations. Sometimes the diagnostician may ask for videos of the teen in places where she or he is able to speak normally.

Specifically, the diagnosis is based on the teen having the ability to speak in some settings and not in others. For the diagnosis to be confirmed, the inability to speak must interfere with schooling and other social activities that most teens are otherwise able to negotiate easily.

How Is Selective Mutism Treated?

Early intervention is crucial for the successful treatment of SM. The most effective treatment has been shown to be behavioral therapy using controlled exposure. The therapist works with the teen and parents and systematically approaches the settings in which the teen cannot speak. The therapist gradually builds the teen's confidence, one situation at a time, during which she or he is never pressured to speak. Instead, the teen is encouraged with positive reinforcement. The therapist provides the parents with specialized techniques to apply in real-life settings. The predictability and control that therapy gives the teen helps reduce anxiety and improves self-image as a result of the mastery of speaking skills in various settings.

Medication may be prescribed, but this is not required in all cases of SM. However, if conditions are severe, a physician may prescribe antianxiety medications. In addition, a history of similar disorders in the family and lack of response to behavioral therapy and other forms of psychotherapy may prompt the need for pharmacological intervention. In many cases, when medication has been prescribed, teens are better able to deal with exposure tasks in behavior therapy, which can help lead to successful treatment. The classes of medications prescribed for SM include selective serotonin reuptake inhibitors (SSRIs) and other antidepressants. Some teens respond well to SSRIs in the case of anxiety, but they need to be monitored carefully for side effects.

What Are Other Concerns Related to Selective Mutism?

At one time, a common theory held that SM was often closely related to child abuse, but according to the Selective Mutism Foundation, research has since discarded this line of thinking. The suggestion of child abuse is devastating to families, and it has deterred many parents from seeking appropriate help for their teen's SM. Child abuse can cause similar symptoms in teens; it may not be specific to immediate family members but could be due to other teens or adults. It is best to contact appropriate agencies in suspected cases of child abuse.

Selective mutism is sometimes mistaken for autism, since many teens with this disorder also experience speech and language problems. The crucial difference is that those with SM have the ability to speak and function normally in some settings.

Selective mutism is not necessarily limited to children. Most teens who experience SM at a young age do so for a short period, but others may find that it continues over many years. If misdiagnosed or improperly treated, SM could persist into adulthood. Studies have shown that some adults report struggling with the symptoms of SM and having to deal with residual symptoms, such as shyness, social anxiety, depression, and panic attacks for many years.

Parents can help teens with SM by providing them with opportunities to socialize and speak in low-stress settings. They can implement behavioral techniques in all social situations in which the teen finds it difficult to speak. To do this properly, parents should enlist the assistance of school authorities, teachers, school psychologists, guidance counselors, and social workers to implement a consistent treatment plan.

References

1. "Selective Mutism (SM) Basics," Child Mind Institute, n.d.
2. "Understanding Selective Mutism Brochure. A Silent Cry for Help!" Selective Mutism Foundation, n.d.
3. "Selective Mutism," The American Speech-Language-Hearing Association (ASHA), n.d.

CHAPTER 13
SPECIFIC PHOBIAS

About This Chapter: Text in this chapter begins with excerpts from "Phobias," MedlinePlus, National Institutes of Health (NIH), June 12, 2020; Text under the heading "Screening for Specific Phobias" is excerpted from "Specific Phobias," U.S. Department of Veterans Affairs (VA), December 23, 2019.

A phobia is a type of anxiety disorder. It is a strong, irrational fear of something that poses little or no real danger.

There are many specific phobias. Acrophobia is a fear of heights. Agoraphobia is a fear of public places, and claustrophobia is a fear of closed-in places. If you become anxious and extremely self-conscious in everyday social situations, you could have a social phobia. Other common phobias involve tunnels, highway driving, water, flying, animals, and blood.

People with phobias try to avoid what they are afraid of. If they cannot, they may experience:

- Panic and fear
- Rapid heartbeat
- Shortness of breath
- Trembling
- A strong desire to get away

Phobias usually start in children or teens, and continue into adulthood. The causes of specific phobias are not known, but they sometimes run in families.

Treatment helps most people with phobias. Options include medicines, therapy, or both.

> Specific phobia is an intense, irrational fear of something that poses little or no actual danger. Although adults with phobias may realize that these fears are irrational, even thinking about facing the feared object or situation brings on severe anxiety symptoms.

Screening for Specific Phobias

As the name suggests, a person with a specific phobia experiences intense fear in response to an object or situation. For example, fear of blood or needles, fear of enclosed places, and fear of flying are common specific phobias, with fear of spiders, fear of snakes, and fear of heights being most common. While many people describe being very afraid of certain situations or things, they may not be bothered by their fear or it may not stop them from doing things because they do not worry about being faced with the feared situation or object. For example, for a man who lives in New York City, a fear of snakes may not be very concerning to him and it likely does not get in the way of him doing things he needs to do. In this case, the fear would not necessarily be considered a specific phobia and he probably would not have a need for treatment.

If anyone feel very afraid of, or feel a need to avoid, any of the objects or situations below? If the answer is "yes" and then it is found that the fear or avoidance of one or more of these situations is getting in that person way, she or he may consider speaking with a physician or mental-health professional about their concerns.

- Animals (such as snakes, spiders, dogs, insects)
- Driving
- Heights, storms or water
- Enclosed places (such as elevators)
- Blood or needles
- Air travel
- Some other object or situation

CHAPTER 14
AGORAPHOBIA

About This Chapter: Text in this chapter begins with excerpts from "Agoraphobia," National Institute of Mental Health (NIMH), November 1, 2017; Text beginning with the heading "Diagnosis" is excerpted from "Panic Disorder and Agoraphobia?" Mental Illness Research, Education and Clinical Centers (MIRECC), U.S. Department of Veterans Affairs (VA), August 12, 2016. Reviewed August 2020.

Agoraphobia is an anxiety disorder that involves intense fear and anxiety of any place or situation where escape might be difficult. Agoraphobia involves avoidance of situations such as being alone outside of the home; traveling in a car, bus, or airplane; or being in a crowded area.

Lifetime Prevalence of Agoraphobia among Adolescents

- Based on diagnostic interview data from National Comorbidity Survey Adolescent (NCS-A) Supplement, Figure 14.1 shows lifetime prevalence of agoraphobia among U.S. adolescents aged 13 to 18.
- An estimated 2.4 percent of adolescents had agoraphobia at some time during their life, and all had severe impairment.
- The prevalence of agoraphobia among adolescents was higher for females (3.4%) than for males (1.4%).

Diagnosis

To receive a diagnosis of agoraphobia, a person needs to exhibit high levels of fear or anxiety about at least two of the following situations, for at least six months or longer:

1. Using public transportation
2. Being in open spaces, such as parks or on bridges
3. Being in enclosed places such as theaters or stores
4. Being in a crowd or standing in line
5. Being outside of the home alone

A person with a diagnosis of agoraphobia fears or avoids these situations because they are concerned that they will not be able to escape them. Others fear that they

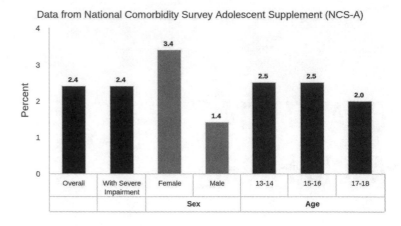

Data from National Comorbidity Survey Adolescent Supplement (NCS-A)

Figure 14.1. Lifetime Prevalence of Agoraphobia among Adolescents (2001–2004)

might not receive help if they develop panic like symptoms or other incapacitating or embarrassing symptoms (such as fear of incontinence or fear of falling in the elderly). The situations almost always cause fear or anxiety in individuals with agoraphobia, and their fears are out of proportion with the actual danger involved in approaching these situations. The fear or avoidance must cause significant distress or impairment in major areas of functioning in order to receive a diagnosis of agoraphobia. If a person is avoiding these situations because of concerns related to a medical condition, the anxiety and avoidance must be clearly excessive.

Finally, to receive a diagnosis of agoraphobia, the clinician must determine that the symptoms are not better explained by another mental-health diagnosis. For example, if the person only avoids social situations, social anxiety disorder might be diagnosed. If they avoid places that remind them of a traumatic event, posttraumatic stress disorder (PTSD) might be diagnosed. Other disorders associated with avoidance, such as major depression, specific phobias, and separation anxiety disorder, might be diagnosed instead of agoraphobia if symptoms are better accounted for by those disorders.

Course of Illness

Between one-third to one-half of people will have panic attacks prior to the onset of agoraphobia; the average age of onset for those individuals is late teens. For those who do not have panic attacks prior to the onset of agoraphobia, the average age of onset is later in the mid- to late-20's. While most develop the disorder at a younger age, a third of individuals will have an onset after age 40. Agoraphobia tends to be a chronic illness if left untreated. Most individuals with agoraphobia also have co-occurring psychiatric disorders, such as anxiety, mood, and/or substance-use disorders.

How Family Members Can Help

Family members of individuals with panic disorder and/or agoraphobia can support their relative's recovery in many ways. It is important for the person who is experiencing anxiety to first visit a medical doctor for a thorough evaluation. If possible, family members could also attend to help answer questions and to provide support. If medication is prescribed, family members can provide support in regularly taking those medications. Family members can also support attendance to psychotherapy appointments by giving reminders and providing transportation to the clinic. If the individual with panic disorder and/or agoraphobia is in therapy, it might be helpful for family members to talk with the therapist to learn specifics about the illness and how they can provide support. Cognitive-behavioral therapy (CBT) includes homework assignments, and family members can encourage their relative to engage in the homework and offer to help, if relevant. For example, family members can help reinforce the concept that panic attacks are not dangerous and work with their relative to consider alternative, nonscary thoughts about the attacks. If the person is engaging in a relaxation or mindfulness practice as part of treatment, family members can help by giving the time and space for their relative to engage in such a practice at home.

Studies have shown that partner-assisted exposure therapy helps reduce symptoms of panic and agoraphobia. Family members can encourage exposure practice with their relative. If there are situations that the person is completely avoiding, family members can offer to initially accompany them into those situations, with the goal being that the person would eventually go into those situations by themselves. Lastly, family members can provide emotional support. Some aspects of panic disorder and agoraphobia can be quite frustrating to relatives. For example, a person with these disorders might avoid making plans, cancel at the last minute for fear of having a panic attack, frequently ask for reassurance about whether or not their symptoms are dangerous, or have difficulty doing things that are easy for most people (e.g., going to the store, driving on the freeway, or going out to restaurants). Family members who understand that these types of behaviors are a part of the disorder may feel less frustration and more warmth and empathy towards their relative.

Treatment
Cognitive-Behavioral Therapy

One of the most effective treatments for panic disorder and agoraphobia is CBT, which can be used alone or in conjunction with medications. CBT can often be utilized effectively on its own for milder cases, whereas a combination is often preferred for more severe cases. CBT is a structured treatment that can be provided in an individual or group format, usually on a weekly basis. There are also some self-help books and manuals that are based on the principles of CBT. The goal of CBT is to significantly reduce or eliminate panic attacks, as well as significantly decrease the fear and behavior changes associated with them. Much of the work of CBT is done between sessions in the form of "homework," so that the person can monitor their panic symptoms and apply the techniques learned in therapy sessions.

Cognitive-behavioral therapy for panic disorder is based on the assumptions that:

1. Individuals with panic disorder misinterpret their panic attacks as dangerous or scary.
2. They are overly attuned to their bodily sensations, making them more vulnerable to experiencing attacks.
3. They often make changes in their behaviors, such as avoidance of situations that they associate with the attacks. One of the goals of treatment is to help the person have a more realistic view of their panic attacks, in order to help make them less scary. This is done through providing education about panic disorder, teaching people to be aware of their scary thoughts about the attacks, and instructing them on how to change these thoughts to make them more realistic and less frightening.

A technique called "interoceptive exposure" is used to help people overcome their fear of the bodily sensations associated with panic attacks. Interoceptive exposure involves engaging in specific exercises to bring on the symptoms of anxiety and panic in a controlled way. Although often uncomfortable at first, these exposure exercises are very effective for alleviating the distress of experiencing symptoms of panic and eventually the symptoms themselves. Finally, CBT utilizes in vivo exposures, in which a person systematically starts to face the people, places, and activities that they might be avoiding as a result of the panic attacks. For example, if someone is avoiding exercising or drinking caffeine for fear of having an attack, the therapist will work with them to strategically plan on introducing and continuing these avoided activities.

With CBT for agoraphobia, the emphasis would likely be on the in vivo exposure element of treatment. By engaging in in vivo exposure therapy, individuals with agoraphobia will systematically and frequently approach feared situations and learn that they are not scary or dangerous.

Relaxation Training

Some therapists use relaxation training as a method of reducing anxiety and panic attacks. It can be used in conjunction with CBT and/or medication, but most professionals agree that relaxation training alone is probably not sufficient to fully alleviate panic symptoms for most people. One type of relaxation strategy often used for panic disorder is diaphragmatic breathing, or belly breathing. This type of breathing, which leads to deeper breaths and more oxygen in the lungs, might be particularly helpful for those who experience shortness of breath, chest pain, or dizziness during their panic attacks. Diaphragmatic breathing is also a relaxation strategy for treating more generalized anxiety, which might then reduce one's susceptibility to having a panic attack. Likewise, progressive muscle relaxation, a type of relaxation which involves tensing and relaxing different muscles in the body, can also lead to reducing generalized anxiety.

Mindfulness and Acceptance Practices

Mindfulness is another technique often used in conjunction with CBT and/or medication. Contrary to what some people think, mindfulness and relaxation are not the same thing, although many people find practicing mindfulness to be relaxing. There are many ways to practice mindfulness. One common way is to sit quietly and focus attention on one's breath, without actually trying to change the breath. People who regularly practice mindfulness can learn to be less reactive to their emotions and changes in their bodies. They can learn to be more accepting of negative emotional states, such as anxiety. For those with panic disorder and agoraphobia, mindfulness can teach people to observe their anxiety, rather than feeding into it with negative thoughts and avoidance behaviors. Thus, acceptance of one's anxiety can cause the anxiety to lessen and feel less scary.

Medications

- There are different types of medications that are very effective for panic disorder and agoraphobia. These include antidepressant medications, benzodiazepines, and anticonvulsants.
- These medications work by modulating gamma-aminobutyric acid (GABA), serotonin, norepinephrine, or dopamine—neurotransmitters believed to regulate anxiety and mood.
- Sometimes the medication you first try may not lead to the improvements you desire with regard to your anxiety. What works well for one person may not do as well for another. Be open to trying another medication or combination of medications in order to find a good fit. Let your doctor know if your symptoms have not improved and do not give up searching for the right medication!
- All medications may cause side effects, but many people have no side effects or minor side effects. The side effects people typically experience are tolerable and subside in a few days. Check with your doctor if any of the common side effects listed persist or become bothersome. In rare cases, these medications can cause severe side effects. Contact your doctor immediately if you experience one or more severe symptoms.

Antidepressant Medications

- Antidepressant medications, while initially developed for depression, have been found to be successful in treating anxiety disorders and are commonly used to treat panic disorder. While many available antidepressants are listed here, the evidence for their effectiveness in treating panic disorder varies considerably. You should discuss medication choices with your doctor.
- Antidepressant medications work to increase the following neurotransmitters: serotonin, norepinephrine, and/or dopamine.

- Antidepressants must be taken as prescribed for three to four weeks before you can expect to see positive changes in your symptoms. So do not stop taking your medication because you think it is not working. Give it time!
- Once you have responded to treatment, it is important to continue treatment. It is typical for treatment to continue for 6 to 9 months. Discontinuing treatment earlier may lead to a relapse of symptoms. If you have a more severe case of panic disorder, the doctor might recommend long-term treatment.
- To prevent the panic disorder from coming back or worsening, do not abruptly stop taking your medications, even if you are feeling better. Stopping your medication can cause a relapse. Medication should only be stopped under your doctor's supervision. If you want to stop taking your medication, talk to your doctor about how to correctly stop it.
- When taking antidepressant medications for panic disorder, if you forget to take a dose, a safe rule of thumb is: If you missed your regular time by three hours or less, you should take that dose when you remember it. If it is more than three hours after the dose should have been taken, just skip the forgotten dose and resume your medication at the next regularly scheduled time. Never double up on doses of your antidepressant to "catch up" on those you have forgotten.

CHAPTER 15
SOCIAL ANXIETY DISORDER

About This Chapter: This chapter includes text excerpted from "Social Anxiety Disorder: More Than Just Shyness," National Institute of Mental Health (NIMH), December 21, 2016. Reviewed August 2020.

Are you extremely afraid of being judged by others?

Are you very self-conscious in everyday social situations?

Do you avoid meeting new people?

If you have been feeling this way for at least six months and these feelings make it hard for you to do everyday tasks—such as talking to people at work or school—you may have a social anxiety disorder.

Social anxiety disorder (also called "social phobia") is a mental-health condition. It is an intense, persistent fear of being watched and judged by others. This fear can affect work, school, and your other day-to-day activities. It can even make it hard to make and keep friends. But social anxiety disorder does not have to stop you from reaching your potential. Treatment can help you overcome your symptoms.

What Is Social Anxiety Disorder?

Social anxiety disorder is a common type of anxiety disorder. A person with social anxiety disorder feels symptoms of anxiety or fear in certain or all social situations, such as meeting new people, dating, being on a job interview, answering a question in class, or having to talk to a cashier in a store. Doing everyday things in front of people—such as eating or drinking in front of others or using a public restroom—also causes anxiety or fear. The person is afraid that she or he will be humiliated, judged, and rejected.

The fear that people with social anxiety disorder have in social situations is so strong that they feel it is beyond their ability to control. As a result, it gets in the way of going to work, attending school, or doing everyday things. People with social anxiety disorder may worry about these and other things for weeks before they happen. Sometimes, they end up staying away from places or events where they think they might have to do something that will embarrass them.

Some people with the disorder do not have anxiety in social situations but have performance anxiety instead. They feel physical symptoms of anxiety in situations such as giving a speech, playing a sports game, or dancing or playing a musical instrument on stage.

Social anxiety disorder usually starts during youth in people who are extremely shy. Social anxiety disorder is not uncommon; research suggests that about 7 percent of Americans are affected. Without treatment, social anxiety disorder can last for many years or a lifetime and prevent a person from reaching her or his full potential.

What Are the Signs and Symptoms of Social Anxiety Disorder?

When having to perform in front of or be around others, people with social anxiety disorder tend to:

- Blush, sweat, tremble, feel a rapid heart rate, or feel their "mind going blank"
- Feel nauseous or sick to their stomach
- Show a rigid body posture, make little eye contact, or speak with an overly soft voice
- Find it scary and difficult to be with other people, especially those they do not already know, and have a hard time talking to them even though they wish they could
- Be very self-conscious in front of other people and feel embarrassed and awkward
- Be very afraid that other people will judge them
- Stay away from places where there are other people

What Causes Social Anxiety Disorder

Social anxiety disorder sometimes runs in families, but no one knows for sure why some family members have it while others do not. Researchers have found that several parts of the brain are involved in fear and anxiety. Some researchers think that misreading of others' behavior may play a role in causing or worsening social anxiety. For example, you may think that people are staring or frowning at you when they truly are not. Underdeveloped social skills are another possible contributor to social anxiety. For example, if you have underdeveloped social skills, you may feel discouraged after talking with people and may worry about doing it in the future. By learning more about fear and anxiety in the brain, scientists may be able to create better treatments. Researchers are also looking for ways in which stress and environmental factors may play a role.

How Is Social Anxiety Disorder Treated?

First, talk to your doctor or healthcare professional about your symptoms. Your doctor should do an exam and ask you about your health history to make sure that an unrelated physical problem is not causing your symptoms. Your doctor may refer you to a mental-health specialist, such as a psychiatrist, psychologist, clinical social worker, or counselor. The first step to effective treatment is to have a diagnosis made, usually by a mental-health specialist.

Social anxiety disorder is generally treated with psychotherapy (sometimes called "talk" therapy), medication, or both. Speak with your doctor or healthcare provider about the best treatment for you. If your healthcare provider cannot provide a referral, visit the NIMH Help for Mental Illnesses web page at www.nimh.nih.gov/findhelp for resources you may find helpful.

Psychotherapy

A type of psychotherapy called "cognitive-behavioral therapy" (CBT) is especially useful for treating social anxiety disorder. CBT teaches you different ways of thinking, behaving, and reacting to situations that help you feel less anxious and fearful. It can also help you learn and practice social skills. CBT delivered in a group format can be especially helpful.

Support Groups

Many people with social anxiety also find support groups helpful. In a group of people who all have social anxiety disorder, you can receive unbiased, honest feedback about how others in the group see you. This way, you can learn that your thoughts about judgment and rejection are not true or are distorted. You can also learn how others with social anxiety disorder approach and overcome the fear of social situations.

Medications

There are three types of medications used to help treat social anxiety disorder:

- Antianxiety medications
- Antidepressants
- Beta-blockers

Antianxiety medications are powerful and begin working right away to reduce anxious feelings; however, these medications are usually not taken for long periods of time. People can build up a tolerance if they are taken over a long period of time and may need higher and higher doses to get the same effect. Some people may even become dependent on them. To avoid these problems, doctors usually prescribe antianxiety medications for short periods, a practice that is especially helpful for older adults.

Antidepressants are mainly used to treat depression, but are also helpful for the symptoms of social anxiety disorder. In contrast to antianxiety medications, they may take several weeks to start working. Antidepressants may also cause side effects, such as headaches, nausea, or difficulty sleeping. These side effects are usually not severe for most people, especially if the dose starts off low and is increased slowly over time. Talk to your doctor about any side effects that you have.

Beta-blockers are medicines that can help block some of the physical symptoms of anxiety on the body, such as an increased heart rate, sweating, or tremors. Beta-blockers are commonly the medications of choice for the "performance anxiety" type of social anxiety.

Your doctor will work with you to find the best medication, dose, and duration of treatment. Many people with social anxiety disorder obtain the best results with a combination of medication and CBT or other psychotherapies.

Do not give up on treatment too quickly. Both psychotherapy and medication can take some time to work. A healthy lifestyle can also help combat anxiety. Make sure to get enough sleep and exercise, eat a healthy diet, and turn to family and friends who you trust for support.

CHAPTER 16
PANIC DISORDERS

About This Chapter: Text beginning with the heading "Overwhelming Fear" is excerpted from "Panic Disorder: When Fear Overwhelms," National Institute of Mental Health (NIMH), 2016. Reviewed August 2020; Text under the heading "Prevalence of Panic Disorder among Adolescents" is excerpted from "Panic Disorder," National Institute of Mental Health (NIMH), November 2017.

Overwhelming Fear

Do you sometimes have sudden attacks of anxiety and overwhelming fear that last for several minutes? Maybe your heart pounds, you sweat, and you feel like you cannot breathe or think. Do these attacks occur at unpredictable times with no obvious trigger, causing you to worry about the possibility of having another one at any time?

If so, you may have a type of anxiety disorder called "panic disorder." Left untreated, panic disorder can lower your quality of life because it may lead to other fears and mental-health disorders, problems at work or school, and social isolation.

What Is It like to Have Panic Disorder?

"One day, without any warning or reason, a feeling of terrible anxiety came crashing down on me. I felt like I could not get enough air, no matter how hard I breathed. My heart was pounding out of my chest, and I thought I might die. I was sweating and felt dizzy. I felt like I had no control over these feelings and like I was drowning and could not think straight.

"After what seemed like an eternity, my breathing slowed and I eventually let go of the fear and my racing thoughts, but I was totally drained and exhausted. These attacks started to occur every couple of weeks, and I thought I was losing my mind. My friend saw how I was struggling and told me to call my doctor for help."

What Is Panic Disorder?

People with panic disorder have sudden and repeated attacks of fear that last for several minutes or longer. These are called "panic attacks." Panic attacks are characterized by a fear of disaster or of losing control even when there is no real danger. A person

Panic disorder is an anxiety disorder characterized by unexpected and repeated episodes of intense fear accompanied by physical symptoms that may include chest pain, heart palpitations, shortness of breath, dizziness, or abdominal distress. These episodes occur "out of the blue," not in conjunction with a known fear or stressor.

(Source: "Panic Disorder," National Institute of Mental Health (NIMH))

may also have a strong physical reaction during a panic attack. It may feel like having a heart attack. Panic attacks can occur at any time, and many people with panic disorder worry about and dread the possibility of having another attack.

A person with panic disorder may become discouraged and feel ashamed because she or he cannot carry out normal routines like going to school or work, going to the grocery store, or driving.

Panic disorder often begins in the late teens or early adulthood. More women than men have panic disorder. But, not everyone who experiences panic attacks will develop panic disorder.

What Causes Panic Disorder

Panic disorder sometimes runs in families, but no one knows for sure why some family members have it while others do not. Researchers have found that several parts of the brain, as well as biological processes, play a key role in fear and anxiety. Some researchers think that people with panic disorder misinterpret harmless bodily sensations as threats. By learning more about how the brain and body functions in people with panic disorder, scientists may be able to create better treatments. Researchers are also looking for ways in which stress and environmental factors may play a role.

What Are the Signs and Symptoms of Panic Disorder?

People with panic disorder may have:
- Sudden and repeated panic attacks of overwhelming anxiety and fear
- A feeling of being out of control, or a fear of death or impending doom during a panic attack
- Physical symptoms during a panic attack, such as a pounding or racing heart, sweating, chills, trembling, breathing problems, weakness or dizziness, tingly or numb hands, chest pain, stomach pain, and nausea
- An intense worry about when the next panic attack will happen
- A fear or avoidance of places where panic attacks have occurred in the past

How Is Panic Disorder Treated?

First, talk to your doctor about your symptoms. Your doctor should do an exam and ask you about your health history to make sure that an unrelated physical problem is not causing your symptoms. Your doctor may refer to you a mental-health specialist, such as a psychiatrist or psychologist.

Panic disorder is generally treated with psychotherapy, medication, or both. Talk with your doctor about the best treatment for you.

Psychotherapy. A type of psychotherapy called "cognitive-behavioral therapy" (CBT) is especially useful as a first-line treatment for panic disorder. CBT teaches you different ways of thinking, behaving, and reacting to the feelings that come on with a panic attack. The attacks can begin to disappear once you learn to react differently to the physical sensations of anxiety and fear that occur during panic attacks.

Medication. Doctors also may prescribe different types of medications to help treat panic disorder:

- Selective serotonin reuptake inhibitors (SSRIs)
- Serotonin-norepinephrine reuptake inhibitors (SNRIs)
- Beta-blockers
- Benzodiazepines

The SSRIs and SNRIs are commonly used to treat depression, but they are also helpful for the symptoms of panic disorder. They may take several weeks to start working. These medications may also cause side effects, such as headaches, nausea, or difficulty sleeping. These side effects are usually not severe for most people, especially if the dose starts off low and is increased slowly over time. Talk to your doctor about any side effects that you have.

Another type of medication called "beta-blockers" can help control some of the physical symptoms of panic disorder, such as rapid heart rate. Although doctors do not commonly prescribe beta-blockers for panic disorder, they may be helpful in certain situations that precede a panic attack.

Benzodiazepines, which are sedative medications, are powerfully effective in rapidly decreasing panic attack symptoms, but they can cause tolerance and dependence if you use them continuously. Therefore, your doctor will only prescribe them for brief periods of time if you need them.

Your doctor will work with you to find the best medication and dose for you.

For more information about these medications, see www.nimh.nih.gov/health/topics/mental-health-medications. Also check the U.S. Food and Drug Administration's (FDA) website (www.fda.gov) for the latest information on warnings, patient medication guides, or newly approved medications.

Do not give up on treatment too quickly. Both psychotherapy and medication can take some time to work. A healthy lifestyle can also help combat panic disorder. Make sure to get enough sleep and exercise, eat a healthy diet, and turn to family and friends who you trust for support.

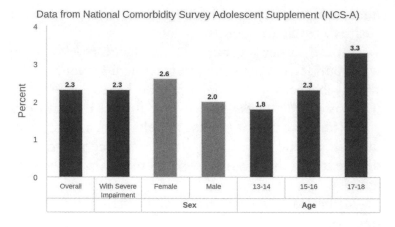

Data from National Comorbidity Survey Adolescent Supplement (NCS-A)

Figure 16.1. Lifetime Prevalence of Panic Disorder among Adolescents (2001–2004)

Prevalence of Panic Disorder among Adolescents

- Based on diagnostic interview data from the National Comorbidity Survey Adolescent (NCS-A) Supplement, Figure 16.1 shows lifetime prevalence of panic disorder among U.S. adolescents aged 13 to 18.
  - An estimated 2.3 percent of adolescents had panic disorder, and 2.3 percent had severe impairment. *Diagnostic and Statistical Manual of Mental Disorders, Fourth Edition* (*DSM-IV*) criteria were used to determine impairment.
  - The prevalence of panic disorder among adolescents was higher for females (2.6%) than for males (2.0%).

CHAPTER 17
DISRUPTIVE MOOD DYSREGULATION DISORDER

About This Chapter: This chapter includes text excerpted from "Disruptive Mood Dysregulation Disorder," National Institute of Mental Health (NIMH), January 2017.

Disruptive mood dysregulation disorder (DMDD) is a childhood condition of extreme irritability, anger, and frequent, intense temper outbursts. DMDD symptoms go beyond being a "moody" child—children with DMDD experience severe impairment that requires clinical attention. DMDD is a fairly new diagnosis, appearing for the first time in the *Diagnostic and Statistical Manual of Mental Disorders* (*DSM-5*), published in 2013 (www.psychiatry.org/psychiatrists/practice/dsm).

Signs and Symptoms of Disruptive Mood Dysregulation Disorder
Disruptive mood dysregulation disorder symptoms typically begin before the age of 10, but the diagnosis is not given to children under 6 or adolescents over 18. A child with DMDD experiences:
- Irritable or angry mood most of the day, nearly every day
- Severe temper outbursts (verbal or behavioral) at an average of three or more times per week that are out of keeping with the situation and the child's developmental level
- Trouble functioning due to irritability in more than one place (e.g., home, school, with peers)

To be diagnosed with DMDD, a child must have these symptoms steadily for 12 or more months.

Risk Factors of Disruptive Mood Dysregulation Disorder

It is not clear how widespread DMDD is in the general population, but it is common among children who visit pediatric mental-health clinics. Researchers are exploring risk factors and brain mechanisms of this disorder.

Treatment and Therapies of Disruptive Mood Dysregulation Disorder

Disruptive mood dysregulation disorder is a new diagnosis. Therefore, treatment is often based on what has been helpful for other disorders that share the symptoms of irritability and temper tantrums. These disorders include attention deficit hyperactivity disorder (ADHD), anxiety disorders, oppositional defiant disorder, and major depressive disorder.

If you think your child has DMDD, it is important to seek treatment. DMDD can impair a child's quality of life and school performance and disrupt relationships with her or his family and peers. Children with DMDD may find it hard to participate in activities or make friends. Having DMDD also increases the risk of developing depression or anxiety disorders in adulthood.

While researchers are still determining which treatments work best, two major types of treatment are currently used to treat DMDD symptoms:

- Medication
- Psychological treatments
  - Psychotherapy
  - Parent training
  - Computer-based training

Psychological treatments should be considered first, with medication added later if necessary, or psychological treatments can be provided along with medication from the beginning.

It is important for parents or caregivers to work closely with the doctor to make a treatment decision that is best for their child.

Medications

Many medications used to treat children and adolescents with mental illness are effective in relieving symptoms. However, some of these medications have not been studied in depth and/or do not have the U.S. Food and Drug Administration (FDA) approval for use with children or adolescents. All medications have side effects and the need for continuing them should be reviewed frequently with your child's doctor.

Stimulants

Stimulants are medications that are commonly used to treat ADHD. There is evidence that, in children with irritability and ADHD, stimulant medications also decrease irritability.

Stimulants should not be used in individuals with serious heart problems. According to the FDA, people on stimulant medications should be periodically monitored for change in heart rate and blood pressure.

Antidepressants

Antidepressant medication is sometimes used to treat the irritability and mood problems associated with DMDD. Ongoing studies are testing whether these medicines are effective for this problem. It is important to note that, although antidepressants are safe and effective for many people, they carry a risk of suicidal thoughts and behavior in children and teens. A "black box" warning—the most serious type of warning that a prescription can carry—has been added to the labels of these medications to alert parents and patients to this risk. For this reason, a child taking an antidepressant should be monitored closely, especially when they first start taking the medication.

Atypical Antipsychotic

An atypical antipsychotic medication may be prescribed for children with very severe temper outbursts that involve physical aggression toward people or property. Risperidone and aripiprazole are FDA-approved for the treatment of irritability associated with autism and are sometimes used to treat DMDD. Atypical antipsychotic medications are associated with many significant side-effects, including suicidal ideation/behaviors, weight gain, metabolic abnormalities, sedation, movement disorders, hormone changes, and others.

Psychological Treatments

Psychotherapy

Cognitive-behavioral therapy (CBT), a type of psychotherapy, is commonly used to teach children and teens how to deal with thoughts and feelings that contribute to their feeling depressed or anxious. Clinicians can use similar techniques to teach children to more effectively regulate their mood and to increase their tolerance for frustration. The therapy also teaches coping skills for regulating anger and ways to identify and relabel the distorted perceptions that contribute to outbursts. Other research psychotherapies are being explored at the National Institute of Mental Health (NIMH).

Parent Training

Parent training aims to help parents interact with a child in a way that will reduce aggression and irritable behavior and improve the parent-child relationship. Multiple studies show that such interventions can be effective. Specifically, parent training teaches parents more effective ways to respond to irritable behavior, such as anticipating events that might lead a child to have a temper outburst and working ahead to avert the outburst. Training also focuses on the importance of predictability, being consistent with children, and rewarding positive behavior.

Computer-Based Training

Evidence suggests that irritable youth with DMDD may be prone to misperceiving ambiguous facial expressions as angry. There is preliminary evidence that computer-based training designed to correct this problem may help youth with DMDD or severe irritability.

CHAPTER 18
MAJOR DEPRESSIVE DISORDER

About This Chapter: This chapter includes text excerpted from "Major Depression," National Institute of Mental Health (NIMH), February 2019.

Major depression is one of the most common mental disorders in the United States. For some individuals, major depression can result in severe impairments that interfere with or limit one's ability to carry out major life activities.

The past-year prevalence data presented here for major depressive episode are from the 2017 National Survey on Drug Use and Health (NSDUH) (www.samhsa.gov/data/sites/default/files/cbhsq-reports/NSDUHDetailedTabs2017/NSDUHDetailedTabs2017.htm#tab8-56A). The NSDUH study definition of major depressive episode is based mainly on the 5th edition of the *Diagnostic and Statistical Manual of Mental Disorders* (*DSM-5*):

- A period of at least two weeks when a person experienced a depressed mood or loss of interest or pleasure in daily activities, and had a majority of specified symptoms, such as problems with sleep, eating, energy, concentration, or self-worth.
- No exclusions were made for a major depressive episode symptoms caused by medical illness, substance-use disorders, or medication.

Prevalence of Major Depressive Episode among Adolescents

- Figure 18.1 shows the past-year prevalence of major depressive episode among U.S. adolescents in 2017.
  - An estimated 3.2 million adolescents aged 12 to 17 in the United States had at least one major depressive episode. This number represented 13.3 percent of the U.S. population aged 12 to 17.
  - The prevalence of major depressive episode was higher among adolescent females (20.0%) compared to males (6.8%).
  - The prevalence of major depressive episode was highest among adolescents reporting two or more races (16.9%).

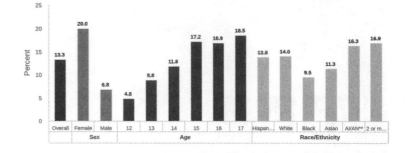

Figure 18.1. Past-Year Prevalence of Major Depressive Episode among U.S. Adolescents (2017)

*All other groups are non-Hispanic or Latinx

**AI/AN = American Indian/Alaska Native

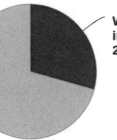

Without severe impairment 29%

With severe impairment 71%

Figure 18.2. Past-Year Severity of Major Depressive Episode among U.S. Adolescents (2017)

Major Depressive Episode with Impairment among Adolescents

- In 2017, an estimated 2.3 million adolescents aged 12 to 17 in the United States had at least one major depressive episode with severe impairment. This number represented 9.4 percent of the U.S. population aged 12 to 17.
- Figure 18.2 shows overall past-year prevalence of major depressive episode with and without severe impairment among U.S. adolescents. Of adolescents with major depressive episode, approximately 70.77 percent had severe impairment.

Treatment of Major Depressive Episode among Adolescents

- Figure 18.3 shows data on treatment received within the past year by U.S. adolescents aged 12 to 17 with major depressive episode in 2017. Treatment types included health professional only, medication only, and combined health professional and medication.

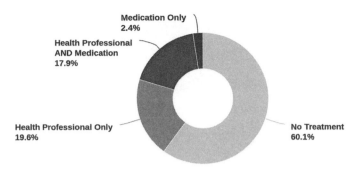

Figure 18.3. Past-Year Treatment Received among Adolescents Major
Depressive Episode (2017)

- An estimated 19.6 percent received care by a health professional alone, and
  another 17.9 percent received combined care by a health professional and
  medication treatment.
- Treatment with medication alone was least common (2.4%).
- Approximately 60.1 percent of adolescents with major depressive episode
  did not receive treatment.

CHAPTER 19
PERSISTENT DEPRESSIVE DISORDER (DYSTHYMIA)

> About This Chapter: Text in this chapter begins with excerpts from "Depressive Disorders in Children and Adolescents," Effective Health Care Program, Agency for Healthcare Research and Quality (AHRQ), October 19, 2017; Text under the heading "Dysthymic Disorder among Children" is excerpted from "Dysthymic Disorder among Children," National Institute of Mental Health (NIMH), November 1, 2017.

Approximately 1 in 10 adolescents aged 13 to 18 has either a major depressive disorder or dysthymic disorder. Depressive disorders negatively impact social and academic outcomes, and are associated with poor long-term outcomes and increased risk of suicide. Some believe that persistent depressive disorder (PDD), or dysthymia, is important to diagnose and manage for children and adolescents since the consequences of PDD are increasingly recognized as grave; and can include severe functional impairment, increased morbidity from physical disease, and increased risk of suicide. Current clinical guidelines recommend the use of psychotherapy with or without antidepressants for children and adolescents with depressive disorders seen in primary and mental healthcare, and outline steps for treating children and adolescents with acute mental health and behavioral problems presenting in EDs. However, there continue to be concerns that antidepressants may be associated with higher rates of suicidality. It is also unclear how nonpharmacological and pharmacological treatments compare to each other, whether certain treatments are

> Persistent depressive disorder (PDD) (formerly "dysthymic disorder") is characterized by chronic low-level depression that is not as severe, but may be lasting longer than major depressive disorder. A diagnosis of persistent depressive disorder requires having experienced a combination of depressive symptoms for two years or more.
>
> *(Source: "Persistent Depressive Disorder (Dysthymic Disorder)," National Institute of Mental Health (NIMH))*

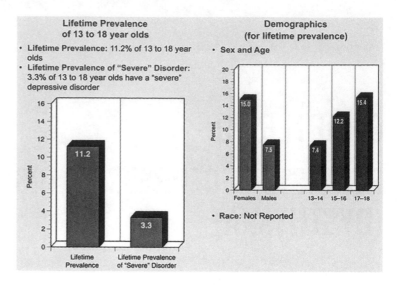

Figure 19.1. Major Depressive Disorder/Dysthymia

more effective for certain population subgroups, and whether early interventions can effectively prevent the development of depressive disorders.

Dysthymic Disorder among Children

Dysthymic disorder is characterized by chronic low-level depression. While the depression is not as severe as that characterizing major depressive disorder, a diagnosis of dysthymia requires having experienced a combination of depressive symptoms for two years or more.

The National Comorbidity Survey—Adolescent (NCS-A) Supplement examines both dysthymic disorder and major depressive disorder together. These depressive disorders have affected approximately 11.2 percent of 13 to 18-year-olds in the United States at some point during their lives. Girls are more likely than boys to experience depressive disorders. Additionally, 3.3 percent of 13 to 18-year-olds have experienced a seriously debilitating depressive disorder.

CHAPTER 20
PREMENSTRUAL DYSPHORIC DISORDER

About This Chapter: This chapter includes text excerpted from "Sex Hormone–Sensitive Gene Complex Linked to Premenstrual Mood Disorder," National Institute of Mental Health (NIMH), January 3, 2017.

Sex Hormone–Sensitive Gene Complex Linked to Premenstrual Mood Disorder

The National Institutes of Health (NIH) researchers have discovered molecular mechanisms that may underlie a woman's susceptibility to disabling irritability, sadness, and anxiety in the days leading up to her menstrual period. Such premenstrual dysphoric disorder (PMDD) affects 2 to 5 percent of women of reproductive age, whereas less severe premenstrual syndrome (PMS) is much more common.

"We found dysregulated expression in a suspect gene complex which adds to evidence that PMDD is a disorder of cellular response to estrogen and progesterone," explained Peter Schmidt, M.D. of the NIH's National Institute of Mental Health (NIMH), Behavioral Endocrinology Branch. "Learning more about the role of this gene complex holds hope for improved treatment of such prevalent reproductive endocrine-related mood disorders."

Schmidt, David Goldman, M.D., of the NIH's National Institute on Alcohol Abuse and Alcoholism (NIAAA), and colleagues, report on their findings January 3, 2017, in the journal Molecular Psychiatry.

Premenstrual dysphoric disorder (PMDD) is a health problem that is similar to premenstrual syndrome (PMS), but is more serious. PMDD causes severe irritability, depression, or anxiety in the week or two before your period starts. Symptoms usually go away two to three days after your period starts. You may need medicine or other treatment to help with your symptoms.

(Source: "Premenstrual Dysphoric Disorder (PMDD)," Office on Women's Health (OWH), U.S. Department of Health and Human Services (HHS))

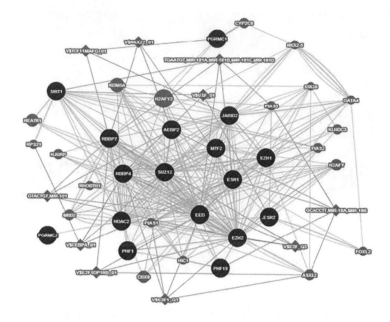

Figure 20.1. ESC or E(Z) Gene Network *(Source: Peter Schmidt, M.D., National Institute of Mental Health (NIMH), David Goldman, M.D., National Institute on Alcohol Abuse and Alcoholism (NIAAA))*
Expression of this ESC/E(Z) gene network was found to be systematically disturbed in PMDD.

"This is a big moment for women's health, because it establishes that women with PMDD have an intrinsic difference in their molecular apparatus for response to sex hormones—not just emotional behaviors they should be able to voluntarily control," said Goldman.

By the late 1990s, the NIMH team had demonstrated that women who regularly experience mood disorder symptoms just prior to their periods were abnormally sensitive to normal changes in sex hormones—even though their hormone levels were normal. But, the cause remained a mystery.

In women with PMDD, experimentally turning off estrogen and progesterone eliminated PMDD symptoms, while experimentally adding back the hormones triggered the reemergence of symptoms. This confirmed that they had a biologically-based behavioral sensitivity to the hormones that might be reflected in molecular differences detectable in their cells.

Following up on clues—including the fact that PMS is 56 percent heritable—the NIH researchers studied the genetic control of gene expression in cultured white blood cell lines from women with PMDD and controls. These cells express many of the same genes expressed in brain cells—potentially providing a window into genetically-influenced differences in molecular responses to sex hormones.

An analysis of all gene transcription in the cultured cell lines turned up a large gene complex in which gene expression differed conspicuously in cells from patients compared to controls. Notably, this ESC/E(Z) (Extra Sex Combs/Enhancer of Zeste) gene complex regulates epigenetic mechanisms that govern the transcription of genes into proteins in response to the environment including sex hormones and stressors.

More than half of the ESC/E(Z) genes were over-expressed in PMDD patients' cells, compared to cells from controls. But paradoxically, protein expression of four key genes was decreased in cells from women with PMDD. In addition, progesterone boosted expression of several of these genes in controls, while estrogen decreased expression in cell lines derived from PMDD patients. This suggested dysregulated cellular response to the hormones in PMDD.

"For the first time, we now have cellular evidence of abnormal signaling in cells derived from women with PMDD, and a plausible biological cause for their abnormal behavioral sensitivity to estrogen and progesterone," explained Schmidt.

Using cutting edge "disease in a dish" technologies, the researchers are now following up the leads discovered in blood cell lines in neurons induced from stem cells derived from the blood of PMDD patients—in hopes of gaining a more direct window into the ESC/E(Z) complex's role in the brain.

CHAPTER 21
SUBSTANCE-INDUCED DEPRESSIVE AND ANXIETY DISORDER

About This Chapter: This chapter includes text excerpted from "Substance Use Disorder Treatment for People with Co-Occurring Disorders," Substance Abuse and Mental Health Services Administration (SAMHSA), February 1, 2020.

Depressive Disorders and Substance-Use Disorders

Depressive disorders are highly comorbid with substance-use disorders (SUDs). For instance:

- Presence of a 12-month or lifetime *Diagnostic and Statistical Manual of Mental Disorders, Fifth Edition* (*DSM-5*) drug-use disorder (i.e., a nonalcoholic SUD) is associated with a 1.5 to 1.9 increased odds of having any mood disorder, a 1.3 to 1.5 increased odds of having dysthymia, and a 1.2 to 1.3 increased odds of having major depressive disorder (MDD).
- Twelve-month alcohol-use disorder (AUD) is also associated with an increased risk of MDD and lifetime AUD with persistent depression.
- A lifetime diagnosis of *DSM 5* MDD is more likely to occur in individuals with a history of SUDs (58%); for AUD (41%) than in people with a history of any anxiety disorder (37%) or PD (32%).

People with depression and co-occurring SUDs tend to have more severe mood symptoms (e.g., sleep disturbance, feelings of worthlessness), higher risk of suicidal ideation and suicide attempts, worse functioning, more psychiatric comorbidities, and greater disease burden (including increased mortality) than people with MDD alone. They are less likely than people with MDD alone to receive antidepressants—despite strong evidence supporting the efficacy of antidepressant medication in alleviating mood and even some SUD symptoms.

Addiction counselors may represent a way to reduce lags in adequate depression care in people with depressive disorders and SUDs. Among 3.3 million people who reported both MDEs and SUDs between 2008 to 2014, only 55 percent received services for depression in the previous year. However, people who had received SUD treatment in the past year were 1.5 times more likely to have received depression care than people who had not engaged in SUD treatment (80% versus 50%, respectively) and were 1.6 times more likely to perceive their depressive care as being helpful (48% versus 32%) than people who did not access SUD treatment in the previous 12 months.

Other facts about depression and SUDs that addiction counselors should know include the following:

- Both substance use and discontinuance can be associated with depressive symptoms.
- During the first months of sobriety, many people with SUDs can exhibit symptoms of depression that fade over time and that are related to acute and protracted withdrawal.
- People with co-occurring depressive disorders and SUDs typically use a variety of drugs.
- Recent evidence suggests there is increasing cannabis use with depression, although cannabinoids have not been shown to be effective in self-management of depression. In fact, cannabis may actually worsen the course of MDD and reduce chances of treatment-seeking.

Treatment of Major Depressive Disorder and Substance-Use Disorder

Psychotherapy (e.g., integrated cognitive-behavioral therapy (CBT), group CBT), with or without adjunct antidepressant use, can effectively reduce frequency of substance use and depressive symptoms and improve functioning briefly and over the long term. In a review examining MDD and AUD specifically, treatment as usual supplemented with CBT and motivational interviewing had small but significant effects in improving depression and decreasing alcohol use versus treatment as usual alone or other brief psychosocial interventions.

Substance-Induced Depressive Disorders

The lifetime prevalence of substance-induced depressive disorders in the general community is 0.26 percent. Observed rates among clinical populations are much higher. For instance, in a study of people seeking treatment for co-occurring depressive disorders and SUDs, 24 percent had substance-induced depression; rates varied by substance. Among those with 12-month alcohol dependence, prevalence of substance-induced MDD was 22 percent; for past-year cocaine dependence, 22 percent; and for past-year heroin dependence, nearly 37 percent. In another study of people with SUDs, 60 percent of people with depression had a substance-induced rather than independent depressive disorder. *DSM-5* notes that although about 40 percent of people with AUD develop MDD, only about one-third to one-half are cases of independent depression, meaning as much as 75 percent of occurrences of depressive disorders in the context of AUD could be because of intoxication or withdrawal. Depressive disorders or their symptoms could also be because of the long-term effects of substance use.

Diagnosis of a substance-induced versus independent depressive disorder can be difficult given that many people with SUDs do have mood symptoms, like depressed affect, and intoxication and withdrawal from substances can mirror symptoms of depression. During the first months of abstinence, many people with SUDs may exhibit symptoms of depression that fade over time and are related to acute withdrawal. Because depressive symptoms during withdrawal and early recovery may result from SUDs and not an underlying depression, a period of time should elapse before depression is diagnosed. This does not preclude the importance of addressing depressive symptoms during the early stage of recovery, before diagnosis. Further, even if an episode of depression is substance-induced, that does not mean that it should not be treated. Overall, the process of addiction can result in biopsychosocial disintegration, leading to PDD or depression often lasting from months to years.

Substance-induced mood alterations can result from acute and chronic drug use as well as from drug withdrawal. Substance-induced depressive disorders, most notably acute depression lasting from hours to days, can result from sedative-hypnotic intoxication. Similarly, prolonged or subacute withdrawal, lasting from weeks to months, can cause episodes of depression, and sometimes is accompanied by suicidal ideation or attempts.

Stimulant withdrawal may provoke episodes of depression lasting from hours to days, especially following high-dose, chronic use. Acute stimulant withdrawal generally lasts from several hours to 1 week and is characterized by depressed mood, agitation, fatigue, voracious appetite, and insomnia or hypersomnia (oversleeping). Depression resulting from stimulant withdrawal may be severe and can be worsened by the individual's awareness of substance-use-related adverse consequences. Symptoms of craving for stimulants are likely and suicide is possible. Protracted stimulant withdrawal often includes sustained episodes of anhedonia (absence of pleasure) and lethargy with frequent ruminations and dreams about stimulant use.

Stimulant cessation may be followed for several months by bursts of dysphoria, intense depression, insomnia, and agitation. These symptoms may be either worsened or lessened depending on the provider's treatment attitudes, beliefs, and approaches. It is a delicate balance—between allowing time to observe the direction of symptoms to treating the client's presenting symptoms regardless of origin.

Substance-Induced Anxiety Disorders

The prevalence of substance-induced anxiety disorders in the community is unreported and thought to be quite low (less than 0.1%), although likely higher in clinical samples.

Licit and illicit substances can cause symptoms that are identical to those in anxiety. In addition, many medications, toxins, and medical procedures can cause or are associated with an eruption of anxiety. Moreover, these reactions vary greatly from mild manifestations of short-lived symptoms to full-blown manic and other psychotic reactions, which are not necessarily short-lived.

Symptoms that look like anxiety may appear either during use or withdrawal. Alcohol, amphetamine and its derivatives, cannabis, cocaine, hallucinogens, intoxicants, and phencyclidine and its relatives have been reported to cause the symptoms of anxiety during intoxication. Withdrawal from alcohol, cocaine, illicit opioids, and also caffeine and nicotine can also cause manifestations of anxiety. Similarly, withdrawal from depressants, opioids, and stimulants invariably includes potent anxiety symptoms.

PART 3 | DIAGNOSIS AND TREATMENT FOR ANXIETY AND DEPRESSION

CHAPTER 22

CHILDREN AND MENTAL HEALTH: IS THIS JUST A STAGE?

About This Chapter: This chapter includes text excerpted from "Children and Mental Health—Is This Just a Stage?" National Institute of Mental Health (NIMH), June 30, 2018.

When to Seek Help

Even under the best of circumstances, it can be hard to tell the difference between challenging behaviors and emotions that are consistent with typical child development and those that are cause for concern. It is important to remember that many disorders like anxiety, attention deficit hyperactivity disorder and depression, do occur during childhood. In fact, many adults who seek treatment reflect back on how these disorders affected their childhood and wish that they had received help sooner. In general, if a child's behavior persists for a few weeks or longer, causes distress for the child or the child's family, and interferes with functioning at school, at home, or with friends, then consider seeking help. If a child's behavior is unsafe, or if a child talks about wanting to hurt herself or himself or someone else, then seek help immediately.

Young children may benefit from an evaluation and treatment if they:

- Have frequent tantrums or are intensely irritable much of the time
- Often talk about fears or worries
- Complain about frequent stomachaches or headaches with no known medical cause
- Are in constant motion and cannot sit quietly (except when they are watching videos or playing videogames)
- Sleep too much or too little, have frequent nightmares, or seem sleepy during the day
- Are not interested in playing with other children or have difficulty making friends
- Struggle academically or have experienced a recent decline in grades

- Repeat actions or check things many times out of fear that something bad may happen

Older children and adolescents may benefit from an evaluation if they:
- Have lost interest in things that they used to enjoy
- Have low energy
- Sleep too much or too little, or seem sleepy throughout the day
- Are spending more and more time alone, and avoid social activities with friends or family
- Fear gaining weight, or diet or exercise excessively
- Engage in self-harm behaviors (e.g., cutting or burning their skin)
- Smoke, drink, or use drugs
- Engage in risky or destructive behavior alone or with friends
- Have thoughts of suicide
- Have periods of highly elevated energy and activity, and require much less sleep than usual
- Say that they think someone is trying to control their mind or that they hear things that other people cannot hear

First Steps for Parents

If you are concerned about your child, where do you begin?
- Talk with your child's teacher. What is the child's behavior like in school, daycare, or on the playground?
- Talk with your child's pediatrician. Describe the behavior, and report what you have observed and learned from talking with others.
- Ask for a referral to a mental-health professional who has experience and expertise dealing with children.

Finding Answers

An evaluation by a health professional can help clarify problems that may be underlying a child's behavior and provide reassurance or recommendations for next steps. It provides an opportunity to learn about a child's strengths and weaknesses and determine which interventions might be most helpful.

A comprehensive assessment of a child's mental health includes the following:
- An interview with parents addressing a child's developmental history, temperament, relationships with friends and family, medical history, interests, abilities, and any prior treatment. It is important to get a picture of the child's current situation, for example: has she or he changed schools recently, has there been an illness in the family, or a change with an impact on the child's daily life.

- Information gathering from school, such as standardized tests, reports on behavior, capabilities, and difficulties
- An interview with the child about her or his experiences, as well as testing and behavioral observations, if needed

Treatment Options

Assessment results may suggest that a child's behavior is related to changes or stresses at home or school; or is the result of a disorder for which treatment would be recommended. Treatment recommendations may include:

- **Psychotherapy ("Talk therapy").** There are many different approaches to psychotherapy, including structured psychotherapies directed at specific conditions. Information about types of psychotherapies is available on the National Institute of Mental Health (NIMH) Psychotherapies page (www.nimh.nih.gov; search term: psychotherapies). Effective psychotherapy for children always includes:
  - Parent involvement in the treatment (especially for children and adolescents)
  - Teaching skills and practicing skills at home or at school (between session "homework assignments")
  - Measures of progress (e.g., rating scales, improvements on homework assignments) that are tracked over time
- **Medications.** Medication may be used along with psychotherapy. As with adults, the type of medications used for children depends on the diagnosis and may include antidepressants, stimulants, mood stabilizers, and others. General information on specific classes of medications is available on the NIMH's mental-health medications page (www.nimh.nih.gov; search term: medications). Medications are often used in combination with psychotherapy. If different specialists are involved, treatment should be coordinated.
- **Family counseling.** Including parents and other members of the family in treatment can help families understand how a child's individual challenges may affect relationships with parents and siblings and vice versa.
- **Support for parents.** Individual or group sessions that include training and the opportunity to talk with other parents can provide new strategies for supporting a child and managing difficult behavior in a positive way. The therapist can also coach parents on how to deal with schools.

To find information about treatment options for specific disorders, visit www.nimh.nih.gov/health.

Choosing a Mental-Health Professional

It is especially important to look for a child mental-health professional who has training and experience treating the specific problems that your child is experiencing. Ask the following questions when meeting with prospective treatment providers:

- Do you use treatment approaches that are supported by research?
- Do you involve parents in the treatment? If so, how are parents involved?
- Will there be homework between sessions?
- How will progress from treatment be evaluated?
- How soon can we expect to see progress?
- How long should treatment last?

Working with the School

If your child has behavioral or emotional challenges that interfere with her or his success in school, she or he may be able to benefit from plans or accommodations that are provided under laws originally enacted to prevent discrimination against children with disabilities. The health professionals who are caring for your child can help you communicate with the school. A first step may be to ask the school whether an individualized education program or a 504 plan is appropriate for your child. Accommodations might include simple measures such as providing a child with a tape recorder for taking notes, permitting flexibility with the amount of time allowed for tests, or adjusting seating in the classroom to reduce distraction. There are many sources of information on what schools can and, in some cases, must provide for children who would benefit from accommodations and how parents can request evaluation and services for their child:

- There are Parent Training and Information Centers (PTIs) and Community Parent Resource Centers (CPRCs) throughout the United States. The Center for Parent Information and Resources (www.parentcenterhub.org/find-your-center) website lists centers in each state.
- The U.S. Department of Education (ED) (www.ed.gov) has detailed information on laws that establish mechanisms for providing children with accommodations tailored to their individual needs and aimed at helping them succeed in school. The ED also has a website on the Individuals with Disabilities Education Act (IDEA) (sites.ed.gov/idea), and the ED's Office of Civil Rights (OCR) (www2.ed.gov/about/offices/list/ocr/frontpage/pro-students/disability-pr.html) has information on other federal laws that prohibit discrimination based on disability in public programs, such as schools.
- Many of the organizations listed in this brochure as additional resources also offer information on working with schools as well as other more general information on disorders affecting children.

The following organizations and agencies have information on mental-health issues in children. Some offer guidance for working with schools and finding health professionals:

- American Academy of Child and Adolescent Psychiatry (AACAP) (www.aacap.org)
- Association for Behavioral and Cognitive Therapies (ABCT) (www.abct.org/Home/index.cfm)
- Society for Clinical Child and Adolescent Psychology (SCCAP) (sccap53.org)
- EffectiveChildTherapy.org (effectivechildtherapy.org)
- Centers for Disease Control and Prevention (CDC) (www.cdc.gov). See the Children's Mental Health page (www.cdc.gov/childrensmentalhealth/symptoms.html).
- Children and Adults with Attention Deficit/Hyperactivity Disorder (CHADD) (chadd.org)
- Depression and Bipolar Support Alliance (DBSA) (www.dbsalliance.org)
- Interagency Autism Coordinating Committee (IACC) (iacc.hhs.gov)
- International OCD Foundation (IOCDF) (iocdf.org)
- Mental Health America (MHA) (www.mhanational.org)
- National Alliance on Mental Illness (NAMI) (www.nami.org/Home)
- National Association of School Psychologists (NASP) (www.nasponline.org/about school psychology/families-and-educators)
- National Federation of Families for Children's Mental Health (NFFCMH) (www.ffcmh.org)
- Stopbullying.gov (www.stopbullying.gov)
- Substance Abuse and Mental Health Services Administration (SAMHSA) Behavioral Health Treatment Services Locator (findtreatment.samhsa.gov)
- Tourette Association of America (TAA) (tourette.org)

CHAPTER 23

SCREENING AND DIAGNOSTIC TOOLS FOR ANXIETY DISORDERS AND DEPRESSION

About This Chapter: "Screening and Diagnostic Tools for Anxiety Disorders and Depression," © 2020 Omnigraphics. Reviewed August 2020.

Emotional disruption experienced in a person's life can lead to other mental-health problems such as addiction or substance-abuse disorders. So it is quite essential to appropriately diagnose and treat anxiety disorders and depression when the early onset of symptoms manifests. Studies show that approximately 50 percent of adolescents live with undiagnosed or untreated depression. The following are the initial steps to be taken for diagnosing an anxiety disorder or depression syndrome:

1. **Find a psychiatrist.** Seek a mental-health professional for receiving therapy and medications. It is important to do proper research on whether the psychologist's personality and treatment philosophy match your needs. You can also request your primary physician to provide a referral to find a suitable psychiatrist.

2. **Get a psychological evaluation.** Once a therapy session is scheduled, the psychiatrist will ask a few general questions to cover your experience of anxiety and depression symptoms. This is done to identify the level and specific type of anxiety or depression, and it also eliminates the possibility of other mental-health problems such as schizophrenia and posttraumatic stress disorder (PTSD).

3. **Undergo physical exam.** Behavioral and emotional symptoms often indicate an underlying physical condition that has to be treated differently from a mood disorder (differential diagnosis). Anxiety disorders are known to present a differential diagnosis more often than any other mood disorder. For instance, caffeine or substances such as illicit drugs can cause symptoms of anxiety disorders. Also, hyperthyroidism, multiple sclerosis, and various types of cancer are often associated with depression.

There are various screening and diagnostic tests used for assessing anxiety disorders and clinical depression. Once the underlying physical problems have been ruled out by a physician, your psychiatrist may provide specific psychological tests to understand the specific details of your anxiety disorder or depression.

Diagnostic Criteria for Anxiety Disorders

According to the *Diagnostic and Statistical Manual of Mental Disorders, 5th edition* (DSM-V), the criteria for classifying anxiety disorder is defined as follows:

- Excessive worry and anxiety occurs during most days for at least a period of six months, during several occasions or activities, including work or school performance.
- The subject of worry may often shift focus and becomes too challenging to control.
- The anxiety and worry are related to three or more of the six symptoms given below:
  1. Feeling of restlessness
  2. Fatigue
  3. Having trouble concentrating
  4. Irritability
  5. Tensed muscles
  6. Difficulty falling asleep or sleep disturbance

A teen suffering from an anxiety disorder experiences at least a few of the above-mentioned symptoms for more than the past six months.

Screening and Diagnostic Tools for Anxiety Disorders

The following are a few tools used to evaluate anxiety disorders in teens:

GAD-7

The Generalized Anxiety Disorder 7 (GAD-7) is a self-administered test that comprises of seven questions for screening generalized anxiety disorder (GAD). It is generally used in outpatient and primary-care settings to check the severity of the patient's anxiety over the past two weeks. However, it is necessary to undergo clinical assessment and further evaluation to confirm a diagnosis of GAD.

SCARED

Screen for Child Anxiety Related Emotional Disorders, or SCARED, is a screening tool intended for adolescents aged 9 to 18 years and their parents. The SCARED is a self-reported screening questionnaire that can differentiate between anxiety and depression and many other distinct anxiety disorders. It is mostly used as a preliminary diagnostic technique for GAD, social anxiety disorder, phobic disorders, and school anxiety problems. It consists of several anxiety disorder criteria given in *DSM-V* by the American Psychiatric Association (APA).

Some of the other commonly used tools for screening and diagnosing anxiety disorders include:

- Beck Anxiety Inventory (BAI)
- Clinician-Administered PTSD Scale (CAPS)
- Hamilton Anxiety Scale (HAM-A)
- Panic and Agoraphobia Scale (PAS)
- Panic Disorder Severity Scale (PDSS)
- PTSD Symptom Scale—Self-Report Version
- Social Phobia Inventory (SPIN)
- Trauma Screening Questionnaire
- Yale-Brown Obsessive-Compulsive Scale (Y-BOCS)
- Zung Self-Rating Anxiety Scale

Diagnostic Criteria for Major Depression

A depressive episode usually has symptoms such as anhedonia (lack of interest or pleasure) and fatigue. A diagnosis of depression syndrome is made using a structured interview based on the *DSM-V* criteria. Major depression includes five or more of the following symptoms for two consecutive weeks and shows a noticeable change from a person's previous level of functioning:

- Being in a depressed mood more often
- Noticeable lack of interest in all or most activities
- More than 5 percent of body weight changes within a month, including a decrease or increase in appetite
- Insomnia or hypersomnia, almost every day
- Slowing down of thought process and physical movements
- Fatigue or exhaustion
- Feeling worthless and guilty
- Unable to focus or make decisions
- Repetitive thoughts of death or suicide attempt

Screening and Diagnostic Tools for Depression

Some of the common tools that are used by mental-health professionals to screen for depression syndromes in teenagers are listed below.

PHQ-9

The patient health questionnaire-9 (PHQ-9) is a 9-question assessment given to patients by their primary-care providers to screen them for the presence and severity of depression. A depression diagnosis based on the *DSM-V* criteria can be made using the responses from the PHQ-9. It is a self-reporting questionnaire that can help diagnose depression.

KADS

The Kutcher Adolescent Depression Scale (KADS) assists in the public health and clinical recognition of adolescents at risk for depression. It was developed by researchers and clinicians with expertise in the field of teen depression. The six-item KADS is specially designed for institutions such as schools and primary-care settings. It can be used as a screening tool by trained healthcare providers or educators, including guidance counselors, to evaluate adolescents who appear depressed or in distress.

Other such tools for screening and diagnosing depression include:

- Beck Depression Inventory (BDI)
- Beck Hopelessness Scale
- Edinburgh Postnatal Depression Scale (EPDS)
- Geriatric Depression Scale (GDS)
- Hamilton Rating Scale for Depression (HAM-D)
- Hospital Anxiety and Depression Scale
- Major Depression Inventory (MDI)
- Weinberg Screen Affective Scale (WSAS)
- Montgomery-Åsberg Depression Rating Scale (MADRS)
- Zung Self-Rating Depression Scale

References

1. "Diagnostic Tools for Anxiety and Depression," Thoracic Key, July 14, 2017.
2. "Clinical Tools," TeenMentalHealth, March 4, 2020.
3. "Screening Tools," Made Of Millions Foundation, February 26, 2020.
4. "What Is Anxiety Disorder? How to Diagnose | Testing and Assessment," Sunrise House, April 6, 2020.

CHAPTER 24
SCREENING FOR MENTAL DISORDERS

About This Chapter: This chapter includes text excerpted from "Mental Health Screening," MedlinePlus, National Institutes of Health (NIH), February 26, 2020.

What Is a Mental-Health Screening?

A mental-health screening is an exam of your emotional health. It helps find out if you have a mental disorder. Mental disorders are common. They affect more than half of all Americans at some point in their lives. There are many types of mental disorders. Some of the most common disorders include:

- **Depression and mood disorders.** These mental disorders are different than normal sadness or grief. They can cause extreme sadness, anger, and/or frustration.
- **Anxiety disorders.** Anxiety can cause excessive worry or fear at real or imagined situations.
- **Eating disorders.** These disorders cause obsessive thoughts and behaviors related to food and body image. Eating disorders may cause people to severely limit the amount of food they eat, excessively overeat (binge), or do a combination of both.
- **Attention deficit hyperactivity disorder (ADHD).** ADHD is one of the most common mental disorders in children. It can also continue into adulthood. People with ADHD have trouble paying attention and controlling impulsive behavior.
- **Posttraumatic stress disorder (PTSD).** This disorder can happen after you live through a traumatic life event, such as a war or serious accident. People with PTSD feel stressed and afraid, even long after the danger is over.
- **Substance-abuse and addictive disorders.** These disorders involve excessive use of alcohol or drugs. People with substance-abuse disorders are at risk for overdose and death.

- **Bipolar disorder, formerly called "manic depression."** People with bipolar disorder have alternating episodes of mania (extreme highs) and depression.
- **Schizophrenia and psychotic disorders.** These are among the most serious psychiatric disorders. They can cause people to see, hear, and/or believe things that are not real.

The effects of mental disorders range from mild-to-severe to life-threatening. Fortunately, many people with mental disorders can be successfully treated with medicine and/or talk therapy.

What Is It Used For?

A mental-health screening is used to help diagnose mental disorders. Your primary care provider may use a mental-health screening to see if you need to go to a mental-health provider. A mental-health provider is a healthcare professional who specializes in diagnosing and treating mental-health problems. If you are already seeing a mental-health provider, you may get a mental-health screening to help guide your treatment.

Why Do You Need a Mental-Health Screening?

You may need a mental-health screening if you have symptoms of a mental disorder. Symptoms vary depending on the type of disorder, but common signs may include:
- Excessive worrying or fear
- Extreme sadness
- Major changes in personality, eating habits, and/or sleeping patterns
- Dramatic mood swings
- Anger, frustration, or irritability
- Fatigue and lack of energy
- Confused thinking and trouble concentrating
- Feelings of guilt or worthlessness
- Avoidance of social activities

One of the most serious signs of a mental disorder is thinking about or attempting suicide. If you are thinking about hurting yourself or about suicide, seek help right away. There are many ways to get help. You can:
- Call 911 or your local emergency room
- Call your mental-health provider or other healthcare provider
- Reach out to a loved one or close friend
- Call a suicide hotline. In the United States, you can call the National Suicide Prevention Lifeline at 800-273-TALK (800-273-8255).
- If you are a Veteran, call the Veterans Crisis Line at 800-273-8255 or send a text to 838255.

What Happens during a Mental-Health Screening

Your primary care provider may give you a physical exam and ask you about your feelings, mood, behavior patterns, and other symptoms. Your provider may also order a blood test to find out if a physical disorder, such as thyroid disease, may be causing mental-health symptoms.

During a blood test, a healthcare professional will take a blood sample from a vein in your arm, using a small needle. After the needle is inserted, a small amount of blood will be collected into a test tube or vial. You may feel a little sting when the needle goes in or out. This usually takes less than five minutes.

If you are being tested by a mental-health provider, she or he may ask you more detailed questions about your feelings and behaviors. You may also be asked to fill out a questionnaire about these issues.

Will You Need to Do Anything to Prepare for a Mental-Health Screening?

You do not need any special preparations for a mental-health screening.

Are There Any Risks to Screening?

There is no risk to having a physical exam or taking a questionnaire.

There is very little risk to having a blood test. You may have slight pain or bruising at the spot where the needle was put in, but most symptoms go away quickly.

What Do the Results Mean?

If you are diagnosed with a mental disorder, it is important to get treatment as soon as possible. Treatment may help prevent long-term suffering and disability. Your specific treatment plan will depend on the type of disorder you have and how serious it is.

Is There Anything Else You Need to Know about a Mental-Health Screening?

There are many types of providers who treat mental disorders. The most common types of mental-health providers include:

- **Psychiatrist.** She or he is a medical doctor who specializes in mental health. Psychiatrists diagnose and treat mental-health disorders. They can also prescribe medicine.
- **Psychologist.** She or he is professionally trained in psychology. Psychologists generally have doctoral degrees. But they do not have medical degrees. Psychologists diagnose and treat mental-health disorders. They offer one-on-one counseling and/or group therapy sessions. They cannot prescribe medicine, unless they have a special license. Some psychologists work with providers who are able to prescribe medicine.

- **Licensed clinical social worker (L.C.S.W.).** She or he has a master's degree in social work with training in mental health. Some have additional degrees and training. L.C.S.W.s diagnose and provide counseling for a variety of mental-health problems. They cannot prescribe medicine, but can work with providers who are able to.
- **Licensed professional counselor. (L.P.C.).** Most L.P.C.s have a master's degree. But training requirements vary by state. L.P.C.s diagnose and provide counseling for a variety of mental-health problems. They cannot prescribe medicine, but can work with providers who are able to.

C.S.W.s and L.P.C.s may be known by other names, including therapist, clinician, or counselor.

If you do not know which type of mental-health provider you should see, talk to your primary care provider.

CHAPTER 25
IMPORTANCE OF TREATING CHILDHOOD DEPRESSION

About This Chapter: This chapter includes text excerpted from "FDA: Don't Leave Childhood Depression Untreated," U.S. Food and Drug Administration (FDA), September 10, 2014. Reviewed August 2020.

Every psychological disorder, including depression, has some behavioral components.

Depressed children often lack energy and enthusiasm. They become withdrawn, irritable, and sulky. They may feel sad, anxious, and restless. They may have problems in school, and frequently lose interest in activities they once enjoyed.

Some parents might think that medication is the solution for depression-related problem behaviors. In fact, that is not the case. The U.S. Food and Drug Administration (FDA) has not approved any drugs solely for the treatment of "behavior problems." When the FDA approves a drug for depression—whether for adults or children—it is to treat the illness, not the behavior associated with it.

"There are multiple parts to mental illness, and the symptoms are usually what drug companies study and what parents worry about. But, it is rare for us at the FDA to target just one part of the illness," says Mitchell Mathis, M.D., a psychiatrist who is the Director of FDA's Division of Psychiatry Products.

Depression Is Treatable

The first step to treating depression is to get a professional diagnosis; most children who are moody, grouchy, or feel that they are misunderstood are not depressed and do not need any drugs.

Only about 11 percent of adolescents have a depressive disorder by age 18, according to the National Institute of Mental Health (NIMH). Before puberty, girls and boys have the same incidence of depression. After adolescence, girls are twice as likely to have depression as boys. The trend continues until after menopause. "That is a clue that depression might be hormonal, but so far, scientists have not found out exactly how hormones affect the brain," says child and adolescent psychiatrist Tiffany R. Farchione, M.D., the Acting Deputy Director of FDA's Division of Psychiatry Products.

It is hard to tell if a child is depressed or going through a difficult time because the signs and symptoms of depression change as children grow and their brains develop. Also, it can take time to get a correct diagnosis because doctors might be getting just a snapshot of what is going on with the young patient.

"In psychiatry, it is easier to take care of adults because you have a lifetime of patient experience to draw from, and patterns are more obvious" says Mathis. "With kids, you do not have that information. Because we do not like to label kids with lifelong disorders, we first look for any other reason for those symptoms. And if we diagnose depression, we assess the severity before treating the patient with medications."

Getting the Proper Care

The second step is to decide on a treatment course, which depends on the severity of the illness and its impact on the child's life. Treatments for depression often include psychotherapy and medication. The FDA has approved two drugs—fluoxetine (Prozac) and escitalopram (Lexapro)—to treat depression in children. Prozac is approved for ages 8 and older; Lexapro for kids 12 and older.

"We need more pediatric studies because many antidepressants approved for adults have not been proven to work in kids," Farchione says. "When we find a treatment that has been shown to work in kids, we are encouraged because that drug can have a big impact on a child who does not have many medication treatment options."

The FDA requires that all antidepressants include a boxed warning about the increased risks of suicidal thinking and behavior in children, adolescents and young adults up to age 24. "All of these medicines work in the brain and the central nervous system, so there are risks. Patients and their doctors have to weigh those risks against the benefits," Mathis says.

Depression can lead to suicide. Children who take antidepressants might have more suicidal thoughts, which is why the labeling includes a boxed warning on all antidepressants. But, the boxed warning does not say not to treat children, just to be aware of, and to monitor them for, signs of suicidality.

"A lot of kids respond very well to drugs. Oftentimes, young people can stop taking the medication after a period of stability, because some of these illnesses are not a chronic disorder like a major depression," Mathis adds. "There are many things that help young psychiatric patients get better, and drugs are just one of them."

It is important that patients and their doctors work together to taper off the medications. Abruptly stopping a treatment without gradually reducing the dose might lead to problems, such as mood disturbance, agitation, and irritability.

Depression in children should not be left untreated. Untreated acute depression may get better on its own, but it relapses and the patient is not cured. Real improvement can take six months or more, and may not be complete without treatment. And the earlier the treatment starts, the better the outcome.

"Kids just do not have time to leave their depression untreated," Farchione says. "The social and educational consequences of a lengthy recovery are huge. They could fail a grade. They could lose all of their friends."

Medications help patients recover sooner and more completely.

CHAPTER 26
TREATING ANXIETY DISORDERS

About This Chapter: This chapter includes text excerpted from "Understanding Anxiety Disorders Young Adult," Substance Abuse and Mental Health Services Administration (SAMHSA), May 2017.

What Are the Treatment Approaches?

An anxiety disorder can be managed in many ways. This includes the use of psychotherapy or a combination of prescribed medication and therapy. You should consider various treatment options, along with your family and your healthcare provider. Collaborative decisions should be made based on your own priorities and goals. If you are of consenting age, you may need to provide written consent for parents or caregivers to participate on the treatment team. It is important to talk to your healthcare providers about other types of treatment, such as complementary medicine, as well as programs that can provide additional support related to education, employment, housing, and vocation and career development. It is also important to have good self-care, such as a healthy diet, exercise, sleep, and abstinence from illicit drugs. Understanding your treatment will help you play an active, full role in your recovery.

Medications

Medications (particularly a group of medications called "selective serotonin reuptake inhibitors" or "SSRIs") can help manage many of the symptoms of an anxiety disorder. Each person reacts differently to these medications. For that reason, the prescribing healthcare professional may try different doses and different kinds of medication before finding the most effective approach for you. Finding the best medication and the most effective dose for you may take time. In milder cases of an anxiety disorder, medication may not be necessary, and therapy or lifestyle changes (e.g., smoking cessation, decreased caffeine intake, regular exercise, or mindfulness exercises) may be sufficient to manage symptoms.

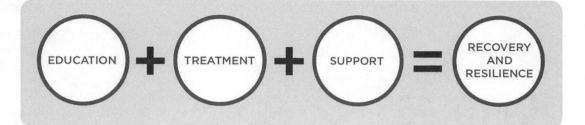

Figure 26.1. Treatment Approach

What Do We Mean by Recovery?
Recovery is a process of change through which individuals improve their health and wellness, live a self-directed life, and strive to reach their full potential. Recovery focuses on wellness and resilience, encouraging [people] to participate actively in their own care.

What Do We Mean by Resilience?
Resilience is the ability to respond to stress, anxiety, trauma, crisis, or disaster. It is critical in recovery [from mental disorders].

Therapy
Behavioral therapy, cognitive-behavioral therapy, or other forms of psychotherapy may be used alone or in combination with medications depending on severity of symptoms. These kinds of treatment build your natural resiliency and provide tools to help understand behaviors that may trigger fear and extreme anxiety.

Support
Your family or peers can also be an important part of your treatment or treatment team for an anxiety disorder. Talking with peers lets you learn from others who are further along in recovery. Family members, caregivers, and peers who are part of your treatment team can help you recognize early symptoms of anxiety before they become a greater problem. These partners can provide important support and encouragement to help you stay focused on your recovery and life goals.

It is important to talk to your healthcare professional about all of your symptoms, such as troublesome fears or phobias, including social situations or insomnia, that may be bothering you. Medications must be taken as prescribed to be effective. Be sure to report any problems or changes to your prescriber, including any use of drugs or medications, smoking, excessive caffeine (energy drinks), or alcohol intake. Sometimes when people try to self-medicate their anxiety with alcohol or drugs, it can get worse. If you have thoughts or plans to harm yourself or others, contact your prescriber or the National Suicide Prevention Lifeline, 800-273-TALK (800-273-8255) or via the web chat function at www.suicidepreventionlifeline.org immediately.

CHAPTER 27
DEPRESSION TREATMENT BASICS

About This Chapter: Text under the heading "How Is Depression Treated?" is excerpted from "Teen Depression," MedlinePlus, National Institutes of Health (NIH), May 3, 2018; Text under the heading "Antidepressant Medications" is excerpted from "Suicidality in Children and Adolescents Being Treated with Antidepressant Medications," U.S. Food and Drug Administration (FDA), February 5, 2018; Text beginning with the heading "Medication Guide for You or Your Family Member's Antidepressant Medicine" is excerpted from "Medication Guide Antidepressant Medicines, Depression and Other Serious Mental Illnesses, and Suicidal Thoughts or Actions," U.S. Food and Drug Administration (FDA), December 4, 2008. Reviewed August 2020.

How Is Depression Treated?

Effective treatments for depression in teens include talk therapy, or a combination of talk therapy and medicines:

Talk Therapy

Talk therapy, also called "psychotherapy" or "counseling," can help you understand and manage your moods and feelings. It involves going to see a therapist, such as a psychiatrist, a psychologist, a social worker, or counselor. You can talk out your emotions to someone who understands and supports you. You can also learn how to stop thinking negatively and start to look at the positives in life. This will help you build confidence and feel better about yourself.

What Is Depression in Teens?

Teen depression is a serious medical illness. It is more than just a feeling of being sad or "blue" for a few days. It is an intense feeling of sadness, hopelessness, and anger or frustration that lasts much longer. These feelings make it hard for you to function normally and do your usual activities. You may also have trouble focusing and have no motivation or energy. Depression can make you feel like it is hard to enjoy life or even get through the day.

There are many different types of talk therapy. Certain types have been shown to help teens deal with depression, including:

- **Cognitive-behavioral therapy (CBT),** which helps you to identify and change negative and unhelpful thoughts. It also helps you build coping skills and change behavioral patterns.
- **Interpersonal therapy (IPT),** which focuses on improving your relationships. It helps you understand and work through troubled relationships that may contribute to your depression. IPT may help you change behaviors that are causing problems. You also explore major issues that may add to your depression, such as grief or life changes.

Programs for Severe Depression

Some teens who have severe depression or are at risk of hurting themselves may need more intensive treatment. They may go into a psychiatric hospital or do a day program. Both offer counseling, group discussions, and activities with mental-health professionals and other patients. Day programs may be full-day or half-day, and they often last for several weeks.

Antidepressant Medications

The FDA directed manufacturers of all antidepressant drugs to revise the labeling for their products to include a boxed warning and expanded warning statements that alert healthcare providers to an increased risk of suicidality (suicidal thinking and behavior) in children and adolescents being treated with these agents, and to include additional information about the results of pediatric studies. The FDA also informed these manufacturers that it has determined that a Patient Medication Guide (MedGuide), which will be given to patients receiving the drugs to advise them of the risk and precautions that can be taken, is appropriate for these drug products. These labeling changes are consistent with the recommendations made to the Agency at a joint meeting of the Psychopharmacologic Drugs Advisory Committee and the Pediatric Drugs Advisory Committee on September 13–14, 2004.

The risk of suicidality for these drugs was identified in a combined analysis of short-term (up to 4 months) placebo-controlled trials of nine antidepressant drugs, including the selective serotonin reuptake inhibitors (SSRIs) and others, in children and adolescents with major depressive disorder (MDD), obsessive-compulsive disorder (OCD), or other psychiatric disorders. A total of 24 trials involving over 4400 patients were included. The analysis showed a greater risk of suicidality during the first few months of treatment in those receiving antidepressants. The average risk of such events on drugs was 4 percent, twice the placebo risk of 2 percent. No suicides occurred in these trials. Based on these data, the FDA has determined that the following points are appropriate for inclusion in the boxed warning:

- Antidepressants increase the risk of suicidal thinking and behavior (suicidality) in children and adolescents with MDD and other psychiatric disorders.
- Anyone considering the use of an antidepressant in a child or adolescent for any clinical use must balance the risk of increased suicidality with the clinical need.
- Patients who are started on therapy should be observed closely for clinical worsening, suicidality, or unusual changes in behavior. Families and caregivers should be advised to closely observe the patient and to communicate with the prescriber.
- A statement regarding whether the particular drug is approved for any pediatric indication(s) and, if so, which one(s).
- Among the antidepressants, only Prozac is approved for use in treating MDD in pediatric patients. Prozac, Zoloft, Luvox, and Anafranil are approved for OCD in pediatric patients. None of the drugs is approved for other psychiatric indications in children.

Pediatric patients being treated with antidepressants for any indication should be closely observed for clinical worsening, as well as agitation, irritability, suicidality, and unusual changes in behavior, especially during the initial few months of a course of drug therapy, or at times of dose changes, either increases or decreases. This monitoring should include daily observation by families and caregivers and frequent contact with the physician. It is also recommended that prescriptions for antidepressants be written for the smallest quantity of tablets consistent with good patient management, in order to reduce the risk of overdose.

In addition to the boxed warning and other information in professional labeling on antidepressants, MedGuides are being prepared for all of the antidepressants to provide information about the risk of suicidality in children and adolescents directly to patients and their families and caregivers. MedGuides are intended to be distributed by the pharmacist with each prescription or refill of a medication.

The FDA plans to work closely with the manufacturers of all approved antidepressant products that are the subject of today's letters to optimize the safe use of these drugs and implement the proposed labeling changes and other safety communications in a timely manner.

Medication Guide for You or Your Family Member's Antidepressant Medicine

This Medication Guide is only about the risk of suicidal thoughts and actions with antidepressant medicines. Talk to your, or your family member's, healthcare provider about:

- All risks and benefits of treatment with antidepressant medicines

- All treatment choices for depression or other serious mental illness

What Is the Most Important Information You Should Know about Antidepressant Medicines, Depression and Other Serious Mental Illnesses, and Suicidal Thoughts or Actions?

- Antidepressant medicines may increase suicidal thoughts or actions in some children, teenagers, and young adults within the first few months of treatment.
- Depression and other serious mental illnesses are the most important causes of suicidal thoughts and actions. Some people may have a particularly high risk of having suicidal thoughts or actions. These include people who have (or have a family history of) bipolar illness (also called "manic-depressive illness") or suicidal thoughts or actions.
- How can you watch for and try to prevent suicidal thoughts and actions in myself or a family member?
  - Pay close attention to any changes, especially sudden changes, in mood, behaviors, thoughts, or feelings. This is very important when an antidepressant medicine is started or when the dose is changed.
  - Call the healthcare provider right away to report new or sudden changes in mood, behavior, thoughts, or feelings.
  - Keep all follow-up visits with the healthcare provider as scheduled. Call the healthcare provider between visits as needed, especially if you have concerns about symptoms.

Call a healthcare provider right away if you or your family member has any of the following symptoms, especially if they are new, worse, or worry you:

- Thoughts about suicide or dying
- Attempts to commit suicide
- New or worse depression
- New or worse anxiety
- Feeling very agitated or restless mood
- Panic attacks
- Trouble sleeping (insomnia)
- New or worse irritability
- Acting aggressive, being angry, or violent
- Acting on dangerous impulses
- An extreme increase in activity and talking (mania)
- Other unusual changes in behavior or mood

What Else Do You Need to Know about Antidepressant Medicines?

- Never stop an antidepressant medicine without first talking to a healthcare provider. Stopping an antidepressant medicine suddenly can cause other symptoms.
- Antidepressants are medicines used to treat depression and other illnesses. It is important to discuss all the risks of treating depression and also the risks of not treating it. Patients and their families or other caregivers should discuss all treatment choices with the healthcare provider, not just the use of antidepressants.
- Antidepressant medicines have other side effects. Talk to the healthcare provider about the side effects of the medicine prescribed for you or your family member.
- Antidepressant medicines can interact with other medicines. Know all of the medicines that you or your family member takes. Keep a list of all medicines to show the healthcare provider. Do not start new medicines without first checking with your healthcare provider.
- Not all antidepressant medicines prescribed for children are FDA-approved for use in children. Talk to your child's healthcare provider for more information.

CHAPTER 28
EXPOSURE THERAPY FOR REDUCING FEAR AND ANXIETY RESPONSES

About This Chapter: "Exposure Therapy for Reducing Fear and Anxiety Responses," © 2020 Omnigraphics. Reviewed August 2020.

Exposure therapy is an effective behavior therapy used for treating fear and anxiety disorders. When people are scared of something, they tend to avoid confronting those objects, situations, or activities as much as possible. Such avoidance behavior may help alleviate fear for a short time, but makes the fear even worse over longer periods of time. Exposure therapy is a psychological technique developed to break this pattern of avoidance in a safe environment where individuals are exposed to the things they fear the most. Around 60–90 percent of people have reported no symptoms or very mild symptoms after completing an exposure therapy course.

Types of Exposure Therapy

Exposure therapy is a vital part of cognitive-behavioral therapy (CBT), and it has been scientifically proven to be helpful for a range of problems, including:
- Social anxiety disorder (SAD)
- Phobic disorders
- Panic disorder (PD)
- Posttraumatic stress disorder (PTSD)
- Obsessive-compulsive disorder (OCD)

There are several variations of exposure therapy that are practiced by psychologists, depending on the format that is best suited for an individual's specific disorder:
- **In vivo exposure.** This involves directly confronting a phobia or situation that causes fear and anxiety in real life. For instance, a person with social anxiety may be instructed to give a speech in front of an audience, or someone with a fear of cats will work towards handling a real cat.

- **Imaginal exposure.** The therapist instructs an individual to vividly imagine or recount the specific situation for their anxiety or fear. Exposure to a picture or memory of the feared object or circumstance, alongside talk therapy can help reduce feelings of distress.
- **Virtual reality or computer-aided exposure.** With increased technological advances, exposure to objects and situations in a realistic computer simulation such as virtual reality is becoming more prevalent. This is done to tackle fears that are impractical to replicate using in vivo exposure. For instance, fear of flying or fear of heights.
- **Interoceptive exposure.** It focuses on inducing physical sensations that are associated with panic or distress. For example, an individual with panic disorder might be instructed by the therapist to run in a safe setting to recreate physical responses similar to a panic attack. This enables the body and mind to learn that an increase in heart rate is not associated with a feeling of panic or danger.

The therapist may sometimes set the pace of the exposure therapy based on the hierarchy of the patient's fears or anxieties:

- **Graded exposure.** This is done by recreating scenarios that a person finds most challenging, starting from the least scary situation. This helps a person to build the confidence required to overcome more significant fears gradually. For example, fear of snakes can be dealt with by looking at pictures of snakes, followed by seeing a snake behind glass, and then eventually holding the snake.
- **Flooding.** The psychologist begins the therapy by exposing the patient to a prolonged and intense version of their most challenging fear. This type of therapy is not practiced widely, but it usually requires only one or two flooding sessions to resolve an issue.
- **Systematic desensitization.** Exposure therapy can also be combined with relaxation exercises to make it more manageable. It helps associate a feeling of calmness with the object or situation that causes worry or anxiety. Systematic desensitization, also known as "graduated exposure therapy" uses relaxation methods to help cope with each fear as a person goes up their hierarchy of fears.
- **Exposure with response prevention (ERP).** It consists of exposure to anxiety-inducing thoughts or circumstances and preventing a neutralizing response. For instance, if a person is afraid of overcrowded buses, they can slowly introduce the patient to more crowded buses and encourage the patient to do nothing to avoid or reduce their feeling of anxiety. This enables the patient to get habituated to the fear and anxiety caused by the trigger situation until these feelings fade away.

Exposure Therapy at Home

It is recommended to get exposure therapy done by a certified mental-health professional since they can alleviate the level of anxiety and ensure that you do not quit halfway through. If the level of anxiety increases and the exposure is stopped, anxiety will be experienced again, and exposure therapy will be more difficult to administer. However, it is possible to perform exposure therapy at home by following the given steps:

- Learn about your specific phobia or anxiety as much as possible using the Internet and other sources to understand the root cause of the disorder or phobia.
- Make a list of ways to gradually lower the anxiety caused due to specific issues, such as thinking or looking at pictures and videos of anxiety-inducing things. Phobia can be overcome by touching or staying in the same room with the thing that causes fear.
- It is helpful having someone hold you accountable or make sure you stop when you experience too much anxiety.
- It is necessary to learn relaxation techniques so you can continue exposure to the trigger until it no longer causes fear or anxiety. A few effective methods include deep breathing, yoga, and progressive muscle relaxation.
- Once you begin the exposure therapy, you cannot stop until the fear or anxiety-provoking trigger no longer affects you. For example, if you are looking at pictures of spiders, do not see the next one until the feeling of anxiety disappears while looking at the first picture. However, if you feel dizzy or have a panic attack, you can take a break before proceeding.
- As soon as you find yourself not anxious or scared of some part of the stimulus, you can stop and try again the next day. Keep repeating the process until you are not afraid or anxious about the trigger anymore.
- It is essential to test yourself further and continue exposure therapy to make sure you do not experience anxious feelings or panic attacks in the future. For example, panic attacks that cause hyperventilation can be prevented by hyperventilating on purpose to make sure the brain gets accustomed to that feeling.

If you are concerned that you may experience a severe reaction to these exposures, it is better to request a psychiatrist's help. People with medical conditions such as a heart problem may also require the help of a medical professional.

References

1. Sissons, Beth. "Exposure Therapy: What It Is and What to Expect," Healthline Media, May 5, 2020.

2. "What Is Exposure Therapy," American Psychological Association (APA), July 15, 2017.
3. "Exposure," Psychology Tools, September 24, 2019.
4. Shaikh, Faiq. "How to Perform Exposure Therapy for Anxiety at Home," Calm Clinic, October 28, 2018.

CHAPTER 29
PLAY AND CREATIVE ART THERAPY

Anxiety often has a significant impact on children since they are not always capable of expressing their troubles. This is because they do not possess the verbal skills to describe their feelings, or they are often unsure of how they feel. Art and play therapy can be useful in such cases, providing children with a format that allows them to communicate their feelings effectively. It can help bridge the gap between the therapist and child by removing the language barrier and any other deterrents that prevent the child from sharing. It also helps children who feel afraid to share their suppressed feelings by giving them a safe emotional distance and protective environment away from their anxiety issues.

Art Therapy for Treating Anxiety in Children

This form of therapy is considered a very effective treatment for children with anxiety disorders due to its nonthreatening approach based on creative expression. It is necessary for anxious children to have a sense of safety in their surroundings to create artwork. There are several ways to let the child feel comfortable during an art therapy session, such as establishing that the child's work of art is not to be judged as "good" or "bad." When determining the progress of art therapy, the aesthetic quality and the technique used in the artwork are not considered as essential factors.

Benefits

Art therapy can help children learn more about their anxiety and ways of coping with it. The following are some of the benefits of art therapy for children.

- **Nonverbal communication.** It enables nonverbal communication of thoughts, emotions, and unconscious symbols and images that enables the therapist to gain a deeper understanding of the child's inner thinking.
- **Safe form of expression.** Art reflects the child's internal conflict and helps them externally represent and physically record their experience and

emotions. Art therapy can be considered a safe place to contain the feelings of the child while processing.

- **Creates self-awareness.** Art therapy encourages the child to be creative, self-discover, problem-solve, and resolve conflicts.

Play Therapy for Treating Anxiety in Children

Play therapy is an expressive therapy similar to art therapy that provides a comprehensive view of the current level of a child's functionality. Making use of creative interventions in play therapy recognizes the relationship between body movement and storytelling. When acting out a narrative or portraying a character, the child is immersed in the story, imitating how they play in school or at home. Playing games such as "tea party" or "house" lets children socialize and represent roles that can assist in forming their sense of identity in the future.

Benefits

Play therapy uses the attributes of a child's playtime to expand the therapeutic values of dealing with their anxiety. It can help children develop positive qualities that can help tackle anxiety disorders.

1. **Enhanced social skills.** It enables a child to adapt to new surroundings and improves their social skills by helping them relax.
2. **Assess and control situations.** It can help a child measure and evaluate the level of worry caused by their anxiety and maintain calm during stressful situations.
3. **Cognitive restructuring.** This can be done using specially designed activities to identify and change or overcome a child's anxious thoughts or feelings.
4. **Self-soothing.** This involves teaching a child how to regain their sense of calm using relaxation techniques such as taking deep breaths or through kinesthetic and tactile touch.
5. **Distraction.** This can help the child divert their thinking away from anxious thoughts.
6. **Positive reinforcement.** Constantly praising the child or rewarding them will help them experience a sense of mastery and increased self-esteem since anxious children often feel they are inadequate.

References

1. Wonders, Lynn. "Play Therapy Interventions for Anxiety," Wonders Counselling, July 30, 2018.
2. Messmer, Kaitlin. "Art and Play Therapy for Children with Anxiety," Digital Commons, October 15, 2010.
3. Eddins, Rachel. "Therapy for My Child: What Are Art and Play Therapy?" Eddins Counselling Group, November 21, 2016.

CHAPTER 30
ROLE OF FAMILY THERAPY IN RECOVERY

About This Chapter: This chapter includes text excerpted from "Family Therapy Can Help," Substance Abuse and Mental Health Services Administration (SAMHSA), November 20, 2013. Reviewed August 2020.

When someone is affected by mental illness or addiction, it can affect the entire family. When that person enters treatment, the family's pain and confusion do not just go away. How does any family member move past the damage that has occurred? How does the family as a whole strengthen the ties that hold it together? Family therapy is one answer. It works together with individual therapy for the benefit of all family members.

What Is Family Therapy?

Family therapy is based on the idea that a family is a system of different parts. A change in any part of the system will trigger changes in all the other parts. This means that when one member of a family is affected by a behavioral health disorder such as mental illness or addiction, everyone is affected.

As a result, family dynamics can change in unhealthy ways. Lies and secrets can build up in the family. Some family members may take on too much responsibility, other family members may act out, and some may just shut down.

Sometimes conditions at home are already unhappy before a family member's mental illness or addiction emerges. That person's changing behaviors can throw the family into even greater turmoil.

Often a family remains stuck in unhealthy patterns even after the family member with the behavioral health disorder moves into recovery. Even in the best circumstances, families can find it hard to adjust to the person in their midst who is recovering, who is behaving differently than before, and who needs support.

Family therapy can help the family as a whole recover and heal. It can help all members of the family make specific, positive changes as the person in recovery changes. These changes can help all family members heal from the trauma of mental illness or addiction.

Who Can Attend Family Therapy?

"Family" means a group of two or more people with close and enduring emotional ties. Using this definition, each person in treatment for a behavioral health disorder has a unique set of family members. Therapists do not decide who should be in family therapy. Instead they ask, "Who is most important to you?"

Sometimes members of a family live together, but sometimes they live apart. Either way, if they are considered family by the person in treatment, they can be included in family therapy. Either parents spouses or partners in-laws, siblings, children, elected, chosen, or honorary family members, other relatives, stepparents, stepchildren, foster parents, foster children, godparents, godchildren, blended family members, extended family members, friends, fellow veterans colleagues who care, mentors, mutual-help group members, and sponsors.

When Should Family Therapy Start?

Family therapy is typically introduced after the individual in treatment for mental illness or addiction has made progress in recovery. This could be a few months after treatment starts, or a year or more later.

Timing is important because people new to recovery have a lot to do. They are working to remain stable in their new patterns of behavior and ways of thinking. They are just beginning to face the many changes they must make to stay mentally healthy or to remain sober. They are learning such things as how to deal with urges to fall into old patterns, how to resist triggers and cravings, how to adhere to medication regimens, and how to avoid temptations to rationalize and make excuses. For them to explore family issues at the same time can be too much. It can potentially contribute to relapse into mental illness or substance using behaviors.

Family therapy tends to be most helpful once the person in treatment is fully committed to the recovery process and is ready to make more changes. The person's counselor can advise on the best time to start family therapy.

What Are the Goals of Family Therapy?

There are two main goals in family therapy. One goal is to help everyone give the right kind of support to the family member in behavioral health treatment, so that recovery sticks and relapse is avoided. The other goal is to strengthen the whole family's emotional health, so that everyone can thrive. Specific objectives for family therapy are unique to each family, and these objectives may change over time. The family decides for itself what to focus on, and when.

Is Family Therapy the Same as Family Education?

No, family therapy is more than family education. Many behavioral health programs conduct education sessions for families on such topics as a particular mental illness, drug and alcohol addiction, treatment, relapse, and recovery. Families can use this

Individual in Recovery From Addiction	Individual in Recovery From Mental Illness	Family
Attainment of sobriety	Working with individual therapist to identify treatment goals	The family system is unbalanced, but healthy change is possible
Adjustment to sobriety	Working through various aspects of the treatment plan (e.g., actively engaging in therapy sessions, taking medications as prescribed, doing therapy "homework")	The family works on developing a new system
Long-term maintenance of sobriety	Termination of treatment after goals have been achieved and a maintenance plan has been established	The family stabilizes a new and healthier lifestyle

Figure 30.1. Stages of Recovery

Distrust	→	Reconciliation
Guilt	→	Forgiveness
Stress	→	Strength
Frustration	→	Understanding
Despair	→	Hope
Sadness	→	Support
Anger	→	Peace
Conflict	→	Agreement
Crisis	→	Resolution

Figure 30.2. Family Therapy Objectives

information to better understand what is happening, how it might affect them, and what to do to help the family member in treatment.

Education is important, but many families also need help applying the information they have learned. Family therapy provides a safe and neutral space in which everyone learns how to adjust to life with a member recovering from mental illness or addiction. The therapist helps the family make changes so that members support each other and treat each other with respect, stop enabling unhealthy behaviors, and learn to trust each other.

Working with a specially trained therapist, family members take a close look at how they act with one another. They look at whether they are conducting themselves in ways that are hurtful or helpful. Family members learn how to modify their behaviors so that they support the needs of the person in recovery as well as the needs of the whole family, including themselves. They also learn how to better communicate with each other, and they practice new ways of talking, relating, and behaving.

Sometimes, a family has problems that have been hidden behind the drama of mental illness or addiction. These problems rise to the surface once the person with a behavioral health disorder goes into treatment. The family therapist can help the family talk together to resolve concerns and mend relationships. The family therapist can refer members of the family to individual counseling if they need or request it.

Who Conducts Family Therapy Sessions

The leader of a family therapy session may be a licensed family therapist, social worker, psychiatrist, psychologist, counselor, clergy member, or some other type of professional. Whatever the title, the leader must meet the legal and professional requirements for working in family therapy. Special training and skills are required, because family therapy is quite different from one-on-one counseling.

The professional who conducts family therapy sessions may be associated with a center that specializes in this work. Sometimes the professional is on the staff of the behavioral health treatment program where the family member is a client.

It is important that the professional who conducts the sessions be sensitive to the family's unique characteristics. This person does not have to have the same background as the family in terms of culture, race, ethnic group, or any other factor. However, she or he must be respectful and understanding without being judgmental.

Typically, the family is provided with a 24-hour crisis phone number. If there is a family emergency between sessions, counseling professionals who staff the crisis line can provide support.

How Is Family Therapy Organized?

Family therapy involves the entire family meeting together. Sometimes part of the family meets. The family therapist may work one-on-one with a particular family member, in addition to the family sessions, although this is not typical.

Sessions usually last about an hour and take place at a clinic, at the therapist's office, or—less often—in a family member's home. The focus of the session may be on the person in treatment, on another family member, or on the family as a whole. Sessions can be low-key or intense, depending on the purpose of the particular session.

Before starting the first session, the therapist may ask family members to sign a contract. This is a way to show that family members agree to certain behaviors, such as to continue individual treatment or to not interrupt each other. Family members also may be asked to sign a consent form to show that they understand the ground rules for privacy and confidentiality. Usually, everyone including the therapist is expected to respect the privacy of what is said during each session and not share it with anyone outside the group. There are some exceptions to this rule, which will be explained on the consent form and by the therapist.

In the session, the family therapist may ask questions or listen and observe while the others talk. The therapist does this to learn such things as how family members behave and communicate with each other and what the family's strengths and needs are. The particular techniques used by the therapist will depend on the phase of treatment for the member in treatment and the family's readiness for change.

The family therapist may refer the whole family or individual members to extra sources of help. For example, the therapist may encourage family members to go for individual counseling, to join a mutual-help group, or to take classes on topics such as parenting or anger management.

What Happens in a Particular Session

There are many things that can happen in family therapy. A session can be devoted to talking about family concerns and how people are feeling. Family members might use the session to talk about a particular crisis or problem that needs solving. Or, they might want to focus on the changes that have been happening.

Another possible topic for a family therapy session is coping skills, such as how to deal with anger, regret, or sadness. Sometimes just letting out feelings and talking about them in therapy sessions can bring relief, understanding, and healing.

The focus of a session might be on learning how to communicate more effectively with each other. For example, the therapist might coach a family member to speak up, to practice saying "no" to unreasonable demands, or to give a compliment. Family members might be asked to rephrase a statement in a more positive way. The therapist also might help family members improve their listening and observing skills to reduce misunderstanding.

Sometimes the therapist asks family members to do homework before the next session. For example, the therapist might ask family members to watch for nice things that other family members say during the week. The therapist might ask family members to eat a meal together or to do something fun together, like play board games or go bowling. The homework is designed to help family members practice new and healthier ways of behaving with each other.

What If Family Members Are Unwilling to Take Part?

Sometimes family members are unwilling to join family therapy. There are many possible reasons for this:

- **Fear.** They may prefer to have the family unit stay as it is, even if that is painful, rather than take chances with the unknown.
- **Fatigue.** They may be tired of dealing with the issues.
- **Concerns about power.** They may feel that they have an advantage the way things are—or that they do not, but family therapy would not fix it.
- **Distrust.** They may be unwilling to risk speaking frankly with other family members or in front of a therapist.

- **Skepticism.** They may not be convinced that family therapy will be useful, or they may have tried it before and not liked it.

It may help to have the family therapist talk one-on-one with unwilling family members. Together they can identify the reasons for resistance, figure out how to resolve concerns, and discuss the benefits of family therapy.

Sometimes what is needed is simply time. Willing members of the family can choose to get started. Unwilling members can join when they are ready.

Is Family Therapy Effective?

Research suggests that behavioral health treatment that includes family therapy works better than treatment that does not. For people with mental illness, family therapy in conjunction with individual treatment can increase medication adherence, reduce rates of relapse and rehospitalization, reduce psychiatric symptoms, and relieve stress.

For people with addiction, family therapy can help them decide to enter or stay in treatment. It can reduce their risk of dropping out of treatment. It also can reduce their continued use of alcohol or drugs, discourage relapse, and promote long-term recovery.

Family therapy benefits other family members besides the person in treatment. By making positive changes in family dynamics, the therapy can reduce the burden of stress that other family members feel. It can prevent additional family members from moving into drug or alcohol use. Research also shows that family therapy can improve how couples treat each other, how children behave, how the whole family gets along, and how the family connects with its neighbors.

Family therapy is not always easy. There will be struggles for everyone involved, but the outcome is worth it. Family therapy is an effective way to help the person in treatment, while also helping the family as a whole.

CHAPTER 31
TREATMENT FOR COMORBID DISORDERS

About This Chapter: This chapter includes text excerpted from "What Are the Treatments for Comorbid Substance Use Disorder and Mental Health Conditions?" National Institute on Drug Abuse (NIDA), April 2020.

Integrated treatment for comorbid drug-use disorder and mental illness has been found to be consistently superior compared with separate treatment of each diagnosis. Integrated treatment of co-occurring disorders often involves using cognitive-behavioral therapy (CBT) strategies to boost interpersonal and coping skills and using approaches that support motivation and functional recovery.

Patients with comorbid disorders demonstrate poorer treatment adherence and higher rates of treatment dropout than those without mental illness, which negatively affects outcomes. Nevertheless, steady progress is being made through research on new and existing treatment options for comorbidity. In addition, research on implementation of appropriate screening and treatment within a variety of settings, including criminal justice systems, can increase access to appropriate treatment for comorbid disorders.

Treatment of comorbidity often involves collaboration between clinical providers and organizations that provide supportive services to address issues such as homelessness, physical health, vocational skills, and legal problems. Communication is critical for supporting this integration of services. Strategies to facilitate effective communication may include co-location, shared treatment plans and records, and case review meetings. Support and incentives for collaboration may be needed, as well as education for staff on co-occurring substance-use and mental-health disorders.

Treatment for Youth

As mentioned previously, the onset of mental illness and substance-use disorders (SUDs) often occurs during adolescence, and people who develop problems earlier typically have a greater risk for severe problems as adults. Given the high prevalence of comorbid mental disorders and their adverse impact on SUD treatment outcomes,

SUD programs for adolescents should screen for comorbid mental disorders and provide treatment as appropriate.

Research indicates that some mental, emotional, and behavioral problems among youth can be prevented or significantly mitigated by evidence-based prevention interventions. These interventions can help reduce the impact of risk factors for SUD and other mental illnesses, including parental unemployment, maternal depression, child abuse and neglect, poor parental supervision, deviant peers, deprivation, poor schools, trauma, limited healthcare, and unsafe and stressful environments. Implementation of policies, programs, and practices that decrease risk factors and increase resilience can help reduce both SUDs and other mental illnesses, potentially saving billions of dollars in associated costs related to healthcare and incarceration.

Other evidence-based interventions emphasize strengthening protective factors to enhance young people's well-being and provide the tools to process emotions and avoid behaviors with negative consequences. Key protective factors include supportive family, school, and community environments.

In addition to the treatment options discussed in this research report, the following treatments have been shown to be effective for children and adolescents:

- **Multisystemic therapy (MST).** This type of therapy targets key factors that are associated with serious antisocial behavior in children and adolescents with SUDs, such as attitudes, family, peer pressure, school, and neighborhood culture.
- **Brief strategic family therapy (BSFT).** This type of therapy targets family interactions that are thought to maintain or exacerbate adolescent SUD and other co-occurring problem behaviors such as conduct problems, oppositional behavior, delinquency, associating with antisocial peers, aggressive and violent behavior, and risky sexual behaviors.
- **Multidimensional family therapy (MDFT).** This therapy is a comprehensive intervention for adolescents which focuses on multiple and interacting risk factors for SUDs and related comorbid conditions. This therapy addresses adolescents' interpersonal and relationship issues, parental behaviors, and the family environment. Families receive assistance with navigating school and social service systems, as well as the juvenile justice system if needed. Treatment includes individual and family sessions.

Medications

Effective medications exist for treating opioid, alcohol, and nicotine-use disorders and for alleviating the symptoms of many other disorders. While most have not been well studied in comorbid populations, some medications may help treat multiple problems. For example, bupropion is approved for treating depression and nicotine dependence.

Table 31.1. Pharmacotherapies Used to Treat Alcohol, Nicotine, and Opioid-Use Disorders

Medication	Use	Dosage Form	DEA Schedule	Application
Buprenorphine-Naloxone	Opioid-use disorder	Sublingual or buccal film buprenorphine/naloxone 2mg/0.5mg, 4mg/1mg, 8mg/2mg, and 12mg/3mg Sublingual tablet: buprenorphine/naloxone 1.4mg/0.36mg, 2mg/0.5mg, 2.9/0.71mg, 5.7mg/1.4mg, 8mg/2mg, 8.6mg/2.1mg, 11.4mg/2.9mg Buccal film: buprenorphine/naloxone 2.1mg/0.3mg, 4.2mg/0.7mg, 6.3mg/1mg	CIII	Used for detoxification and maintenance of abstinence for individuals aged 16 or older
Buprenorphine Hydrochloride	Opioid-use disorder	Sublingual tablet: 2mg, 4mg, 8mg, and 12mg Probuphine® implants 80mgx4 implants for a total of 320mg	CIII	This formulation is indicated for treatment of opioid dependence and is preferred for induction. However, it is considered the preferred formulation for pregnant patients, patients with hepatic impairment, and patients with sensitivity to naloxone. It is also used for initiating treatment in patients transferring from methadone, in preference to products containing naloxone, because of the risk of precipitating withdrawal in these patients. For those already stable on low-to-moderate dose buprenorphine. The administration of the implant dosage form requires specific training and must be surgically.
Methadone	Opioid-use disorder	Tablet: 5mg, 10mg Tablet for suspension: 40mg Oral concentrate: 10mg/mL Oral solution: 5mg/5mL, 10mg/5mL Injection: 10mg/mL	CII	Providers using this medication must be linked to a federally certified Opioid Treatment Program. Under federal regulations, it can be used in persons under age 18 at the discretion of an Opioid Treatment Program physician.

Table 31.1. Continued

Medication	Use	Dosage Form	DEA Schedule	Application
Naltrexone	Opioid-use disorder; alcohol-use disorder	Tablets: 25mg, 50mg, and 100mg Extended-release injectable suspension: 380mg/vial	Not scheduled under the Controlled Substances Act	Provided by prescription; naltrexone blocks opioid receptors, reduces cravings, and diminishes the rewarding effects of alcohol and opioids. Extended-release injectable naltrexone is recommended to prevent relapse to opioids or alcohol. The prescriber need not be a physician, but must be licensed and authorized to prescribe by the state.
Acamprosate	Alcohol-use disorder	Delayed-release tablet: 333mg	Not scheduled under the Controlled Substances Act	Provided by prescription; acamprosate is used in the maintenance of alcohol abstinence. The prescriber need not be a physician, but must be licensed and authorized to prescribe by the state.
Disulfiram	Alcohol-use disorder	Tablet: 250mg, 500mg	Not scheduled under the Controlled Substances Act	When taken in combination with alcohol, disulfiram causes severe physical reactions, including nausea, flushing, and heart palpitations. The knowledge that such a reaction is likely if alcohol is consumed acts as a deterrent to drinking.
Nicotine Replacement Therapies	Nicotine-use disorder	Transdermal patches: 7 to 22 mg/day Gum: 18 to 48 mg/day Lozenges: 40 to 80 mg/day Inhalers: Variable dosing Nasal spray: Up to 40 mg/day	Not scheduled under the Controlled Substances Act	Nicotine replacement therapy helps alleviate withdrawal symptoms in the short-term, and patients with severe nicotine-use disorder might benefit from more long-term use.
Bupropion HCl	Nicotine-use disorder	Tablet: 150 mg/day for three days, then increase to 300 mg/day for 7 to 12 weeks	Not scheduled under the Controlled Substances Act	Bupropion HCl is an antidepressant that has also been shown to assist with nicotine cessation, although the mechanism of action is not understood.
Varenicline	Nicotine-use disorder	Tablet: 0.5 mg/day for three days: 0.5 mg twice a day for days 4 to 7; then 1.0 mg twice a day through week 12	Not scheduled under the Controlled Substances Act	Varenicline helps reduce nicotine cravings.

(Source: The Surgeon General's report and National Cancer Institute (NCI), Cigarette Smoking: Health Risks and How to Quit)

Behavioral Therapies

Behavioral treatment (alone or in combination with medications) is a cornerstone to successful long-term outcomes for many individuals with drug-use disorders or other mental illnesses. Several strategies have shown promise for treating specific comorbid conditions.

Cognitive-Behavioral Therapy

Cognitive-behavioral therapy (CBT) is designed to modify harmful beliefs and maladaptive behaviors and shows strong efficacy for individuals with SUDs. CBT is the most effective psychotherapy for children and adolescents with anxiety and mood disorders.

Dialectical Behavior Therapy

Dialectical behavior therapy (DBT) is designed specifically to reduce self-harm behaviors including suicidal attempts, thoughts, or urges; cutting; and drug use. It is one of the few treatments effective for individuals who meet the criteria for borderline personality disorder.

Assertive Community Treatment

Assertive community treatment (ACT) programs integrate behavioral treatments for severe mental illnesses such as schizophrenia and co-occurring SUDs. ACT is differentiated from other approaches to case management through factors such as a smaller caseload size, team management, outreach emphasis, a highly individualized approach, and an assertive approach to maintaining contact with patients.

Therapeutic Communities

Therapeutic communities (TCs) are a common form of long-term residential treatment for SUDs. They focus on the "resocialization" of the individual, often using broad-based community programs as active components of treatment. TCs are appropriate for populations with a high prevalence of co-occurring disorders such as criminal justice-involved persons, individuals with vocational deficits, vulnerable or neglected youth, and homeless individuals. In addition, some evidence suggests that TCs may be helpful for adolescents who have received treatment for substance use and addiction.

Contingency Management or Motivational Incentives

Contingency management (CM) or motivational incentives (MI) is used as an adjunct to treatment. Voucher or prize-based systems reward patients who practice healthy behaviors and reduce unhealthy behaviors, including smoking and drug use. Incentive-based treatments are effective for improving treatment compliance and reducing tobacco and other drug use, and can be integrated into behavioral health treatment programs for people with co-occurring disorders.

Exposure Therapy

Exposure therapy is a behavioral treatment for some anxiety disorders (phobias and posttraumatic stress disorder (PTSD)) that involves repeated exposure to a feared situation, object, traumatic event, or memory. This exposure can be real, visualized, or simulated, and is always contained in a controlled therapeutic environment. The goal is to desensitize patients to the triggering stimuli and help them develop coping mechanisms, eventually reducing or even eliminating symptoms. Several studies suggest that exposure therapy may be helpful for individuals with comorbid PTSD and cocaine-use disorder, although retention in treatment is a challenge.

Integrated Group Therapy

Integrated group therapy (IGT) is a treatment developed specifically for patients with bipolar disorder and SUD, designed to address both problems simultaneously. This therapy is largely based on CBT principles and is usually an adjunct to medication. The IGT approach emphasizes helping patients understand the relationship between the two disorders, as well as the link between thoughts and behaviors, and how they contribute to recovery and relapse.

Seeking Safety

Seeking safety (SS) is a present-focused therapy aimed at treating trauma-related problems (including PTSD) and SUD simultaneously. Patients learn behavioral skills for coping with trauma/PTSD and SUD.

Mobile Medical Application

In 2017, the U.S. Food and Drug Administration (FDA) approved the first mobile medical application to help treat SUDs. The intention is for patients to use it with outpatient therapy to treat alcohol, cocaine, marijuana, and stimulant-use disorders; it is not intended to treat opioid dependence. The device delivers CBT to patients to teach skills that aid in the treatment of SUDs and increase retention in outpatient therapy programs.

CHAPTER 32
COMPLEMENTARY APPROACH TO ANXIETY AND DEPRESSION

About This Chapter: This chapter includes text excerpted from "Anxiety and Complementary Health Approaches: What the Science Says," National Center for Complementary and Integrative Health (NCCIH), August 2020.

Mind and Body Approaches

Acupuncture

Although some studies of acupuncture for anxiety have had positive outcomes, in general, many of the studies on acupuncture for anxiety have been of poor methodological quality or not of statistical significance. In addition, because the research is extremely variable (e.g., number and variety of acupuncture points, frequency of sessions, and duration of treatment), it is difficult to draw firm conclusions about potential benefits.

What Does the Research Show?

- A 2012 review of 32 studies of acupuncture for anxiety found that although there have been some positive outcomes, the generally poor methodological quality, combined with the wide range of outcome measures used, number and variety of points, frequency of sessions, and duration of treatment makes drawing firm conclusions difficult.
- A 2014 meta-analysis of 14 studies involving 1,034 participants on the efficacy of acupuncture in reducing preoperative anxiety found that acupuncture has a statistically significant effect relative to placebo or nontreatment controls, but the sample size was small. The meta-analysis supports the possibility that acupuncture is superior to placebo for preoperative anxiety.

Safety

- Acupuncture is generally considered safe when performed by an experienced practitioner using sterile needles. Reports of serious adverse events related to acupuncture are rare, but include infections and punctured organs.

Massage Therapy

In some studies massage therapy helped to reduce anxiety for people with cancer or other comorbid medical conditions; however, other studies did not find a statistically significant beneficial effect. Little research has been done on massage for anxiety disorders, and results have been conflicting.

What Does the Research Show?

- A 2014 systematic review and meta-analysis of 18 randomized controlled trials involving 950 women with breast cancer did not find any significant effect of massage on anxiety.
- A 2013 randomized controlled trial of 60 cancer patients examined massage therapy for perioperative pain and anxiety in placement of vascular access devices and found that both massage therapy and structured attention proved beneficial for alleviating preoperative anxiety in these patients.
- A 2012 randomized trial involving 152 cardiac surgery patients found that massage therapy significantly reduced the pain, anxiety, and muscular tension and improved relaxation after cardiac surgery.
- Findings from a 2012 randomized controlled trial of 120 primiparous women with term pregnancy suggest that massage is an effective alternative intervention, decreasing pain and anxiety during labor.

Safety

- Massage therapy appears to have few risks if it is used appropriately and provided by a trained massage professional.

Mindfulness Meditation

Meditation therapy is commonly used and has been shown to be of small to modest benefit for people with anxiety-related symptoms. There is some evidence that transcendental meditation may have a beneficial effect on anxiety. However, there is a lack of studies with adequate statistical power in patients with clinically diagnosed anxiety disorders, which makes it difficult to draw firm conclusions about its efficacy for anxiety disorders.

What Does the Research Show?

- A 2017 randomized controlled trial involving 57 participants with generalized anxiety disorder (GAD) found that mindfulness meditation training was associated with a significantly greater decrease in partial work days and decrease in healthcare utilization.
- A 2014 systematic review and meta-analysis of 47 trials with 3,515 participants found that mindfulness meditation programs had moderate evidence of improved anxiety. The reviewers concluded that clinicians should be aware that meditation programs can result in small-to-moderate reductions of multiple negative dimensions of psychological stress.

- A 2012 systematic review and meta-analysis of 36 randomized controlled trials found evidence of some efficacy of meditative therapies in reducing anxiety symptoms; however, most studies included in the analysis measured only improvement in anxiety symptoms, but not anxiety disorders as clinically diagnosed.
- A 2006 Cochrane review of two randomized controlled trials concluded that because of the small number of studies, conclusions could not be drawn about the efficacy of meditation therapy for anxiety disorders.

Safety
- Meditation is generally considered to be safe for healthy people. However, people with physical limitations may not be able to participate in certain meditative practices involving movement.

Relaxation Techniques
Relaxation techniques may reduce anxiety in individuals with chronic medical problems and those who are having medical procedures. However, research demonstrates that conventional psychotherapy, for individuals with GAD, may be more effective than relaxation techniques.

What Does the Research Show?
- A 2014 meta-analysis of a total of 41 studies involving 2,132 participants with GAD found some indications that cognitive-behavioral therapy (CBT) was more effective than relaxation techniques over the long term.
- A 2016 randomized trial of 236 women undergoing large core breast biopsy found that adjunctive self-hypnotic relaxation decreased procedural pain and anxiety.
- A 2012 randomized controlled trial of 39 participants with inflammatory bowel disease found that those who received the relaxation-training intervention showed a statistically significant improvement in anxiety levels as compared to the control group.

Safety
- Relaxation techniques are generally considered safe for healthy people. People with serious physical or mental-health problems should discuss relaxation techniques with their healthcare providers.

Natural Products
Chamomile
There is some research that suggests that a chamomile extract may be helpful for GAD, but the studies are preliminary, and their findings are not conclusive.

What Does the Research Show?

- A 2016 randomized controlled trial involving 179 participants with moderate-to-severe GAD found that chamomile extract produced a clinical meaningful reduction in anxiety symptoms over 8 weeks.
- Results from a 2009 randomized, double-blind, placebo-controlled efficacy and tolerability trial of chamomile extract in 57 patients with mild-to-moderate GAD suggest that chamomile may have modest anxiolytic activity in patients with mild-to-moderate GAD.

Safety

- There have been reports of allergic reactions, including rare cases of anaphylaxis, in people who have consumed or come into contact with chamomile products.
- People are more likely to experience allergic reactions to chamomile if they are allergic to related plants such as ragweed, chrysanthemums, marigolds, or daisies.
- Interactions between chamomile and cyclosporine and warfarin have been reported, and there are theoretical reasons to suspect that chamomile might interact with other drugs as well.

Kava

Kava extract may produce moderately beneficial effects on anxiety symptoms; however, the use of kava supplements has been linked to a risk of severe liver damage.

What Does the Research Show?

- A 2013 randomized controlled trial involving 75 participants with GAD concluded that standardized kava extract may be a moderately effective short-term option for the treatment of GAD.
- A 2011 review of 66 studies of herbal medicine for depression, anxiety, and insomnia found some evidence that kava may produce beneficial effects for anxiety disorders.
- A 2003 Cochrane review of 12 randomized controlled trials found that compared with placebo, kava extract may be an effective symptomatic treatment for anxiety, although the effect size appears small.

Safety

- The use of kava supplements has been linked to a risk of severe liver damage, according to the U.S. Food and Drug Administration (FDA).
- Kava has been associated with several cases of dystonia and may interact with several drugs, including drugs used for Parkinson disease.
- However, a 2013 randomized controlled trial of 75 participants who received kava extract over a 6-week period found no significant differences across groups for liver function tests, nor any significant adverse reactions

associated with kava administration. Long-term safety studies of kava are needed.

Melatonin
There is some research that suggests melatonin may help reduce anxiety in patients who are about to have surgery and may be as effective as standard treatment with midazolam in reducing preoperative anxiety.

What Does the Research Show?
- A 2017 randomized trial involving 80 children undergoing surgery found that melatonin was as effective as midazolam in reducing children's anxiety in both the preoperative room and at induction of anesthesia.
- A 2015 Cochrane review of 12 studies involving 774 participants found that melatonin compared to placebo, given as premedication, reduced preoperative anxiety (measured 50 to 100 minutes after administration) and may reduce postoperative anxiety (6 hours after surgery). The reviewers also found that melatonin may be equally as effective as standard treatment with midazolam in reducing preoperative anxiety.

Safety
- Melatonin supplements appear to be safe when used short-term; less is known about long-term safety.

Lavender
Although some studies of lavender preparations for anxiety have shown some therapeutic effects, in general, many of these studies have been of poor methodological quality.

What Does the Research Show?
- A 2017 meta-analysis of five studies involving 1,165 participants with anxiety diagnoses found Silexan (lavender oil) to be significantly superior to placebo in ameliorating anxiety symptoms independently of diagnosis. The study also found a tendency for greater clinical effect when analyzing separately GAD patients in comparison with all other diagnosis.
- A 2012 systematic review of 15 randomized controlled trials concluded that methodological issues limit the extent to which any conclusions can be drawn regarding the efficacy of lavender for anxiety.

Safety
- When lavender teas and extracts are taken by mouth, they may cause headache, changes in appetite, and constipation.
- Using lavender supplements with sedative medications may increase drowsiness.

CHAPTER 33

TECHNOLOGY AND THE FUTURE OF MENTAL-HEALTH TREATMENT

About This Chapter: This chapter includes text excerpted from "Technology and the Future of Mental Health Treatment," National Institute of Mental Health (NIMH), September 2019.

Technology has opened a new frontier in mental-health support and data collection. Mobile devices like cell phones, smartphones, and tablets are giving the public, doctors, and researchers new ways to access help, monitor progress, and increase understanding of mental well-being.

Mobile mental-health support can be very simple but effective. For example, anyone with the ability to send a text message can contact a crisis center. New technology can also be packaged into an extremely sophisticated app for smartphones or tablets. Such apps might use the device's built-in sensors to collect information on a user's typical behavior patterns. If the app detects a change in behavior, it may provide a signal that help is needed before a crisis occurs. Some apps are stand-alone programs that promise to improve memory or thinking skills. Others help the user connect to a peer counselor or to a healthcare professional.

Excitement about the huge range of opportunities has led to a burst of app development. There are thousands of mental-health apps available in iTunes and Android app stores, and the number is growing every year. However, this new technology frontier includes a lot of uncertainty. There is very little industry regulation and very little information on app effectiveness, which can lead consumers to wonder which apps they should trust.

Before focusing on the state of the science and where it may lead, it is important to look at the advantages and disadvantages of expanding mental-health treatment and research into a mobile world.

The Pros and Cons of Mental-Health Apps

Experts believe that technology has a lot of potential for clients and clinicians alike. A few of the advantages of mobile care include:

- **Convenience.** Treatment can take place anytime and anywhere (e.g., at home in the middle of the night or on a bus on the way to work) and may be ideal for those who have trouble with in-person appointments.
- **Anonymity.** Clients can seek treatment options without involving other people.
- **An introduction to care.** Technology may be a good first step for those who have avoided mental healthcare in the past.
- **Lower cost.** Some apps are free or cost less than traditional care.
- **Service to more people.** Technology can help mental-health providers offer treatment to people in remote areas or to many people in times of sudden need (e.g., following a natural disaster or terror attack).
- **Interest.** Some technologies might be more appealing than traditional treatment methods, which may encourage clients to continue therapy.
- **24-hour service.** Technology can provide round-the-clock monitoring or intervention support.
- **Consistency.** Technology can offer the same treatment program to all users.
- **Support.** Technology can complement traditional therapy by extending an in-person session, reinforcing new skills, and providing support and monitoring.
- **Objective data collection.** Technology can quantitatively collect information such as location, movement, phone use, and other information.

This new era of mental-health technology offers great opportunities but also raises a number of concerns. Tackling potential problems will be an important part of making sure new apps provide benefits without causing harm. That is why the mental-health community and software developers are focusing on:

- **Effectiveness.** The biggest concern with technological interventions is obtaining scientific evidence that they work and that they work as well as traditional methods.
- **For whom and for what.** Another concern is understanding if apps work for all people and for all mental-health conditions.
- **Privacy.** Apps deal with very sensitive personal information so app makers need to be able to guarantee privacy for app users.
- **Guidance.** There are no industry-wide standards to help consumers know if an app or other mobile technology is proven effective.
- **Regulation.** The question of who will or should regulate mental-health technology and the data it generates needs to be answered.

- **Overselling.** There is some concern that if an app or program promises more than it delivers, consumers may turn away from other, more effective therapies.

Current Trends in App Development

Creative research and engineering teams are combining their skills to address a wide range of mental-health concerns. Some popular areas of app development include:

Self-Management Apps

"Self-management" means that the user puts information into the app so that the app can provide feedback. For example, the user might set up medication reminders, or use the app to develop tools for managing stress, anxiety, or sleep problems. Some software can use additional equipment to track heart rate, breathing patterns, blood pressure, etc. and may help the user track progress and receive feedback.

Apps for Improving Thinking Skills

Apps that help the user with cognitive remediation (improved thinking skills) are promising. These apps are often targeted toward people with serious mental illnesses.

Skill-Training Apps

Skill-training apps may feel more like games than other mental-health apps as they help users learn new coping or thinking skills. The user might watch an educational video about anxiety management or the importance of social support. Next, the user might pick some new strategies to try and then use the app to track how often those new skills are practiced.

Illness Management, Supported Care

This type of app technology adds additional support by allowing the user to interact with another human being. The app may help the user connect with peer support or may send information to a trained healthcare provider who can offer guidance and therapy options. Researchers are working to learn how much human interaction people need for app-based treatments to be effective.

Passive Symptom Tracking

A lot of effort is going into developing apps that can collect data using the sensors built into smartphones. These sensors can record movement patterns, social interactions (such as the number of texts and phone calls), behavior at different times of the day, vocal tone and speed, and more. In the future, apps may be able to analyze these data to determine the user's real-time state of mind. Such apps may be able to recognize changes in behavior patterns that signal a mood episode such as mania, depression, or psychosis before it occurs. An app may not replace a mental-health professional, but it may be able to alert caregivers when a client needs additional attention. The goal is to create apps that support a range of users, including those with serious mental illnesses.

Data Collection

Data collection apps can gather data without any help from the user. Receiving information from a large number of individuals at the same time can increase researchers' understanding of mental health and help them develop better interventions.

Research via Smartphone?

Dr. Patricia Areán's pioneering BRIGHTEN study, showed that research via smartphone app is already a reality. The BRIGHTEN study was remarkable because it used technology to both deliver treatment interventions and also to actually conduct the research trial. In other words, the research team used technology to recruit, screen, enroll, treat, and assess participants. BRIGHTEN was especially exciting because the study showed that technology can be an efficient way to pilot test promising new treatments, and that those treatments need to be engaging.

A New Partnership: Clinicians and Engineers

Researchers have found that interventions are most effective when people like them, are engaged, and want to continue using them. Behavioral health apps will need to combine the engineers' skills for making an app easy to use and entertaining with the clinician's skills for providing effective treatment options.

Researchers and software engineers are developing and testing apps that do everything from managing medications to teaching coping skills to predicting when someone may need more emotional help. Intervention apps may help someone give up smoking, manage symptoms, or overcome anxiety, depression, posttraumatic stress disorder (PTSD), or insomnia. While the apps are becoming more appealing and user-friendly, there still is not a lot of information on their effectiveness.

Evaluating Apps

There are no review boards, checklists, or widely accepted rules for choosing a mental-health app. Most apps do not have peer-reviewed research to support their claims, and it is unlikely that every mental-health app will go through a randomized, controlled research trial to test effectiveness. One reason is that testing is a slow process and technology evolves quickly. By the time an app has been put through rigorous scientific testing, the original technology may be outdated.

Currently, there are no national standards for evaluating the effectiveness of the hundreds of mental-health apps that are available. Consumers should be cautious about trusting a program. However, there are a few suggestions for finding an app that may work for you:

- Ask a trusted healthcare provider for a recommendation. Some larger providers may offer several apps and collect data on their use.
- Check to see if the app offers recommendations for what to do if symptoms get worse or if there is a psychiatric emergency.

What Is NIMH's Role in Mental-Health Intervention Technology?

Between FY2009 and FY2015, NIMH awarded 404 grants totaling 445 million for technology-enhanced mental-health intervention grants. These grants were for studies of computer-based interventions designed to prevent or treat mental-health disorders.

National Institute of Mental Health staff actively review and evaluate research grants related to technology. In recent years, these grants focused on:

- Feasibility, efficacy, and effectiveness research
- Technology for disorders such as schizophrenia, HIV, depression, anxiety, autism, suicide, and trauma
- More interventions for cognitive issues, illness management, behavior, and health communication
- Fewer interventions for a personal computer and more interventions for mobile devices
- More engaging ways to deliver therapies or skill development (e.g., interactive formats or game-like approaches)
- Real-time (users exchanging information with peers or professionals as needed)
- Active and passive mobile assessment/monitoring

A significant portion of NIMH funding of these types of technologies is through the Small Business Innovation Research (SBIR) and Small Business Technology Transfer (STTR) programs.

In addition, NIMH created the National Advisory Mental Health Council Workgroup on Opportunities and Challenges of Developing Information Technologies on Behavioral and Social Science Research to track and guide the cutting edge of this rapidly-changing area. In 2017, the workgroup released a report reviewing the opportunities for—and the challenges of—using new information technologies to study human behaviors relevant to the NIMH mission. NIMH's interest in this area of research was further highlighted in a 2018 notice identifying research on digital health technology to advance the assessment, detection, prevention, treatment, and delivery of services for mental-health conditions as a high-priority area for the Institute.

- Decide if you want an app that is completely automated or an app that offers opportunities for contact with a trained person.
- Search for information on the app developer. Can you find helpful information about her or his credentials and experience?
- Beware of misleading logos. The National Institute of Mental Health (NIMH) has not developed and does not endorse any apps. However, some app developers have unlawfully used the NIMH logo to market their products.
- Search the PubMed database (pubmed.ncbi.nlm.nih.gov) offered by National Library of Medicine (NLM). This resource contains articles on a wide range of research topics, including mental-health app development.
- If there is no information about a particular app, check to see if it is based on a treatment that has been tested. For example, research has shown that Internet-based cognitive-behavioral therapy (CBT) is as effective as conventional CBT for disorders that respond well to CBT, like depression, anxiety, social phobia, and panic disorder.
- Try it. If you are interested in an app, test it for a few days and decide if it is easy to use, holds your attention, and if you want to continue using it. An app is only effective if it keeps users engaged for weeks or months.

The Future: What Types of Research Does NIMH Expect in the Future?

Recently, there has been increased interest in:

- Using mobile technology for a wider range of disorders, from mild depression or anxiety to schizophrenia, autism, and suicide
- Developing and refining new interventions, instead of adapting existing interventions to work with new technologies
- Developing technologies that work on any device
- Incorporating face-to-face contact or remote counseling (phone or online) to provide a balance between technology and the "human touch"

PART 4 | STRENGTHENING PROTECTIVE FACTORS AND MENTAL-HEALTH SUPPORT

CHAPTER 34

UNIQUE ISSUES IN EMOTIONAL AND SOCIAL DEVELOPMENT IN ADOLESCENCE

About This Chapter: Text under the heading "Unique Issues in Emotional Development" is excerpted from "Unique Issues in Emotional Development," Office of Adolescent Health (OAH), U.S. Department of Health and Human Services (HHS), August 10, 2018; Text under the heading "General Emotional Changes Adolescents Experience" is excerpted from "Emotional Development," Office of Adolescent Health (OAH), U.S. Department of Health and Human Services (HHS), July 29, 2018; Text under the heading "Unique Issues in Social Development" is excerpted from "Unique Issues in Social Development," Office of Adolescent Health (OAH), U.S. Department of Health and Human Services (HHS), July 2, 2019.

Unique Issues in Emotional Development

Physical changes increase adolescents' capacity for emotional awareness, self-management, and empathy, but emotional development is strongly influenced by context. This means that many aspects of adolescents' lives can influence their emotional development. Among these aspects are:

- **Self-esteem.** How people feel about themselves—or the way they perceive their own talents, characteristics, and life experiences—can affect their sense of their own worth. An adolescent's self-esteem can be influenced by approval from family, support from friends, and personal successes. Research shows that adolescents with a positive self-concept experience greater academic success than do adolescents who lack this quality. Concerns about body image also are common and can provide opportunities for parents, teachers, and other caring adults to teach self-care, offer encouragement, and reinforce a positive body image. For some adolescents, the concern for body image is extreme and—when combined with other warning signs—may indicate an eating disorder. Eating disorders are one type of mental-health problem among adolescents. However, feeling good about oneself does not necessarily protect against risky behaviors. Therefore, it is still important to limit adolescents'

147

exposure to risky situations and empower young people to make healthy choices when they inevitably come across such a situation.

- **Identity formation.** There are many facets to identity formation, which includes developmental tasks such as becoming independent and achieving a sense of competence. Adolescents may question their passions and values, examine their relationships with family and peers, and think about their talents and definitions of success. Identity formation is an iterative process during which adolescents repeatedly experiment with different ideas, friends, and activities. This experimentation is normal and can provide adolescents opportunities to learn more about themselves and others, but it is not always balanced with thoughtfulness or a cognitive ability to consider the consequences of their actions. Although this path to finding one's identity can prove challenging for some families, it also can motivate adolescents to learn about themselves and become more confident in their own, unique identities.

- **Stress.** Adolescents live in a variety of environments and experience a wide range of stressors that affect emotional development. Learning healthy responses to stressful situations is part of normal development, and some stress can even be positive. However, some adolescents face particularly traumatic events, such as experiencing or witnessing physical or sexual abuse, or school violence. Some of these events are prolonged or recurring, such as chronic neglect or being bullied. Some adolescents also have to deal with multiple types of traumatic stress. These more extreme forms of stress, often referred to as "toxic stress," can weaken an adolescent's immune system, resulting in chronic physical health problems and potentially leading to depression, anxiety, and other mental-health disorders. Toxic stress also can lead to stress-related diseases and cognitive impairment in adulthood. Adolescents who experience this form of stress also are more likely to use harmful substances, engage in other risky behaviors, and experience posttraumatic stress disorder (PTSD), a condition in which a person relives a traumatic event through persistent memories or flashbacks and experiences other symptoms such as insomnia, angry outbursts, or feeling tense. However, people respond to stress differently, and a strong support system can help protect adolescents from long-lasting negative effects and create an environment that enables youth to thrive.

General Emotional Changes Adolescents Experience

Healthy emotional development is marked by a gradually increasing ability to perceive, assess, and manage emotions. This is a biological process driven by physical and cognitive changes and heavily influenced by context and environment. During adolescence young people generally become more aware of their own feelings and the feelings of others, but these perceptions may still be tenuous. Adults sometimes expect adolescents to keep their emotions from interfering with performance in school, work, and other activities, but doing so may be challenging in a complex environment. Some adolescents may be excited to take on new challenges as they become more independent, whereas others may need more support to build their confidence. The process of emotional development gives adolescents the opportunity to build skills, discover unique qualities, and develop strengths for optimal health.

Factors that affect how well adolescents navigate this process include:

- **Hormones.** These critical chemicals in the brain that bring about physical changes also affect adolescent's moods and heighten their emotional responses. These characteristics together mean that teens are more easily swayed by emotion and have difficulty making decisions that adults find appropriate. Adolescence also is a time of rapid and sometimes stressful changes in peer relationships, school expectations, family dynamics, and safety concerns in communities. The body responds to stress by activating specific hormones and activities in the nervous system so that the person can respond quickly and perform well under pressure. The stress response kicks in more quickly for adolescents than it does for adults whose brains are fully developed and can moderate a stress response. Not all stressors are bad. Positive experiences such as landing a first job or getting a driver's permit can trigger a stress response that enables adolescents to approach a challenge with alertness and focus.

- **Self-management.** By managing their own emotions, adolescents can establish positive goals and gain foresight into how their emotions can influence their goals and futures. To improve their ability to manage emotions, adolescents must first learn to recognize and describe strong, complex emotions. Although young people learn to describe basic emotions earlier in life, as they get older they develop an ability to truly grasp what emotions are and understand their impact. When adolescents can recognize how they feel, they can choose how they will react to a situation. They also learn to avoid the problems that strong emotions sometimes cause. However, because the brain's frontal lobe—which is responsible for reasoning, planning, and problem-solving as well as emotions—does not fully develop until the mid-twenties, adolescents may find it difficult to manage their emotions and think through the consequences of their actions. Over time and with the support of parents and helpful adults, adolescents can develop the reasoning and abstract thinking skills that enable them to step back, examine their emotions, and consider consequences before acting rashly.

Unique Issues in Social Development

The way adolescents develop socially largely depends on their environment. For example, some youth live in neighborhoods and attend schools where violence is relatively common. These adolescents must develop different coping strategies than do those who live in neighborhoods with more physical security. Some adolescents also experience trauma. These experiences can evoke stress reactions across all developmental areas. Some survivors of trauma have difficulty regulating emotions, sleeping, eating, and acting on or making decisions. In any case, all adolescents need caring adults in their lives who offer them support, provide opportunities for them to test their new skills, and offer guidance on how to be successful. The key role that environment plays in adolescent development means that adolescents of the same age will differ greatly in their ability to handle diverse social situations.

Here are some other factors that differ among adolescents and can affect their social development:

- **Varying rates of physical development.** Adolescents' bodies change and develop at different rates, and this process does not always happen in sync with other areas of development. For instance, those who develop physically at a relatively young age may be seen and treated more like adults or they may end up spending more time with older youth because of how they look, a pattern that increases their potential for engaging in sexual relationships. However, these more mature-looking adolescents may not be emotionally and cognitively ready to handle those new roles. On the other hand, adolescents who develop later may be seen and treated more like young children.

- **Evolving groups of friends.** Acceptance by a peer group is crucial to adolescents, especially those who are younger. Seeking acceptance might spur them to change the way they think, speak, dress, and behave to make them feel they belong to the group. As a result, younger adolescents tend to hang out with peers who are similar to them (e.g., same race, ethnicity, family income, religion, or class schedule). Older adolescents may branch out to other groups as their social worlds diversify and expand.

- **Differing types of peer pressure.** Peer pressure sometimes gets a bad reputation. The stereotype about this pressure stems from perceptions of delinquent and risky behaviors, including sexual activity and substance abuse, which some adolescents think will earn them greater acceptance among their peers. However, peer pressure can be beneficial, and peer relationships can be largely positive. Positive peer groups practice behaviors such as cooperating, sharing, resolving conflicts, and supporting others. The accepted standards, or norms, of positive peer groups can help adolescents build relationship skills, hold favorable views of themselves, and have the confidence to take positive risks.

- **Changing ways to interact.** As with all technologies, using social media carries both potential risks and potential benefits for adolescents. Text messaging, social networking platforms, blogs, email, and instant messaging can help adolescents stay connected to each other, and express who they are to the world. Today's adolescents have such large social networks that it is not uncommon to have virtual friendships with peers they have never met face-to-face. This digital interaction may curtail nonverbal communication and cues that occur in person that are important for developing social skills; but these interactions are still social and meaningful to the adolescents who participate in them. At the same time, technology and social media have also provided a new forum for harassment. In addition to the 20 percent of high school students who reported being bullied in school in the year 2015, another 16 percent reported being bullied online.

CHAPTER 35
PROTECTIVE AND PROMOTIVE FACTORS IN MENTAL HEALTH

About This Chapter: This chapter includes text excerpted from "Promoting Protective Factors for In-Risk Families and Youth: A Guide for Practitioners," Child Welfare Information Gateway, U.S. Department of Health and Human Services (HHS), September 15, 2015. Reviewed August 2020.

Protective factors are conditions or attributes of individuals, families, communities, or the larger society that, when present, promote well-being and reduce the risk for negative outcomes. These factors may "buffer" the effect of risk exposure and help individuals and families negotiate difficult circumstances and fare better in school, work, and life.

Positive long-term outcomes related to health, school success, and successful transitions to adulthood typically do not occur as the result of single interventions. Focusing on protective factors offers a way to track progress by increasing resilience in the short-term and contributing to the development of skills, personal characteristics, knowledge, relationships, and opportunities that offset risk exposure and contribute to improved well-being.

Which Individual Skills and Capacities Can Improve Well-Being for Children and Youth?

At the individual level, the evidence is strongest for the protective nature of self-regulation skills, relational skills, and problem-solving skills.

- **Self-regulation skills.** It refers to a youth's ability to manage or control emotions and behaviors, which can include self-mastery, anger management, character, long-term self-control, and emotional intelligence.
- **Relational skills.** It refers to a youth's ability to form positive bonds and connections (e.g., social competence, being caring, forming prosocial

relationships), and a youth's interpersonal skills (e.g., communication skills and conflict resolution skills).

- **Problem-solving skills.** It refers to a youth's adaptive functioning skills and ability to solve problems.

These three important skills are related to positive outcomes such as resiliency, having supportive friends, positive academic performance, improved cognitive functioning, and better social skills. They are also related to reductions in posttraumatic stress disorder, stress, anxiety, depression, and delinquency. Finally, these skills are related to more satisfaction with out-of-home placements and fewer placement disruptions.

How Can Parents, Guardians, Other Adults, and Peers Contribute to a Child's Well-Being?

For the youth of all ages, the competencies of the parent or guardian include parenting skills (e.g., establishing clear standards and limits, discipline, and proper care) and positive parent-child interactions (e.g., sensitive, supportive, or caring parenting and close relationships between parent and child). These competencies are related to numerous well-being outcomes such as increases in self-esteem, lower risk of antisocial behavior, lower likelihood of running away and teen pregnancy, reductions in child behavior problems, increases in social skills, better psychological adjustment, and reductions in internalizing behaviors. Also, for children in out-of-home care, improvements in parenting competencies have been associated with family reunification.

The Well-Being of Parents and Other Caregivers

The well-being of parents and other caregivers is an important protective factor, especially for younger youth (under the age of 12). The well-being of parents and caregivers primarily refers to the parents' own positive psychological functioning (e.g., lower rates of depression and other mental-health problems of mothers), well-being, and social supports. This protective factor is related to resilience, fewer conduct problems, better social relationships, and better behavioral health outcomes for their children. The presence of a caring adult is particularly important for teens and young adults. These caring adults are often program staff or home visitors, but can also be mentors, advocates, teachers, or extended family members.

Presence of a Caring Adult

The presence of a caring adult is related to numerous positive outcomes, including greater resilience, lower stress, less likelihood of arrest, reductions in homelessness, higher levels of employment, less delinquent conduct, favorable health, less suicidal ideation, reductions in rapid repeat pregnancies, and better outcomes for the children of teen mothers.

Positive Relationships with Peers

Positive relationships with peers are another source of protection and include both support from peers and positive peer norms. Having friendships and support from peers is related to reductions in depressive symptoms, more empathetic parenting attitudes (among teen mothers), and higher self-esteem. The presence of positive peer norms is related to reductions in rapid repeat pregnancies; less alcohol, tobacco and other drug use; lower levels of sexual activity; less antisocial and delinquent behavior; and more success in school. Ensuring that children and youth have positive peers can be achieved by creating groups with positive attitudes and values.

CHAPTER 36
IMPORTANCE OF SCHOOL CONNECTEDNESS

About This Chapter: Text beginning with the heading "Youth Connectedness Is an Important Protective Factor for Health and Well-Being" is excerpted from "Adolescent Connectedness," Centers for Disease Control and Prevention (CDC), August 21, 2019; Text beginning with the heading "Fostering School Connectedness" is excerpted from "Fostering School Connectedness," Centers for Disease Control and Prevention (CDC), July 2009. Reviewed August 2020.

Youth Connectedness Is an Important Protective Factor for Health and Well-Being

Connectedness is an important protective factor for youth that can reduce the likelihood of a variety of health risk behaviors. "Connectedness" refers to a sense of being cared for, supported, and belonging, and can be centered on feeling connected to school, family (i.e., parents and caregivers), or other important people and organizations in their lives. Youth who feel connected at school and home are less likely to experience negative health outcomes related to sexual risk, substance use, violence, and mental health.

In addition, school connectedness (i.e., the belief by students that adults and peers in the school care about them as individuals) has been shown to have positive effects on academic achievement, including having higher grades and test scores, having better school attendance, and staying in school longer.

Adolescent Connectedness Has Lasting Effects

Recently the CDC findings published in *Pediatrics* suggest that youth connectedness also has lasting effects. Youth who feel connected at school and at home were found to be as much as 66 percent less likely to experience health risk behaviors related to sexual health, substance use, violence, and mental health in adulthood.

Fostering School Connectedness

Students feel more connected to their school when they believe that the adults and other students at school not only care about how well they are learning, but also care about them as individuals. Young people who feel connected to school are more likely to succeed academically and make healthy choices.

All school staff, including teachers, principals, counselors, social workers, nurses, aides, librarians, coaches, nutrition personnel, and others, can have an important and positive influence on students' lives. The time, interest, attention, and emotional support they give students can help them learn and stay healthy.

Why Is School Connectedness Important for Students?

School connectedness is an important factor in both health and learning. Students who feel connected to their school are:

- More likely to attend school regularly, stay in school longer, and have higher grades and test scores
- Less likely to smoke cigarettes, drink alcohol, or have sexual intercourse
- Less likely to carry weapons, become involved in violence, or be injured from dangerous activities such as drinking and driving or not wearing seat belts
- Less likely to have emotional problems, suffer from eating disorders, or experience suicidal thoughts or attempts

Strategies and Actions Teachers and Other School Staff Can Take to Increase School Connectedness

Create Processes That Engage Students, Families, and Communities and That Facilitate Academic Achievement

- **Brainstorm and get involved** in taking steps to improve the school climate and students' sense of connectedness to school. Involve diverse groups of school staff, students, and families in these efforts.
- **Help** plan school policies and activities with teams of students, faculty, staff, and parents.
- **Encourage** students to talk openly with school staff and parents. Involve students in parent-teacher conferences, teacher evaluation, curriculum selection committees, and school health teams.

Provide Opportunities for Families to Be Actively Involved in Their Children's Academic and School Life

- **Engage** parents in meaningful ways in school activities, such as school health teams, tutoring, mentoring, or assisting with grant writing. Identify special opportunities for parents with limited resources or scheduling difficulties to participate in or contribute to classroom or extracurricular activities.
- **Seek** opportunities for parents and students to share their culture with others in school.

- **Communicate** regularly with families about school and classroom activities and policies by e-mail, letters, or updates on the school's website.
- **Translate** materials into languages spoken in students' homes.
- **Establish** regular meetings with parents to discuss their children's behavior, grades, and accomplishments. Request interpreters as needed to ensure clear communication and to avoid misunderstandings arising from language barriers.

Provide Students with the Academic, Emotional, and Social Skills They Need to Engage in School

- **Provide** opportunities for students to improve their interpersonal, stress management, and decision-making skills.
- **Foster** critical and reflective thinking, problem solving, and working effectively with others.
- **Allow and encourage** students to identify, label, express, and assess their feelings.
- **Use** classroom and extracurricular activities to explore and discuss empathy, personal strengths, fairness, kindness, and social responsibility.
- **Use** interactive, experiential activities, and help students personalize the information they learn.
- **Encourage** students to be involved in service learning, peer tutoring, classroom chores, teacher assistance, extracurricular activities, sports programs, and creative projects. Provide public recognition for students' accomplishments in these areas.
- **Correct** inaccurate perceptions about what are "normal" behaviors among students. For example, compare the number of students who actually smoke cigarettes or drink alcohol with the perception that "everyone is doing it."
- **Help** students identify their career and personal goals and map out the steps they can take to meet them.

Use Effective Classroom Management and Teaching Methods to Foster a Positive Learning Environment

- **Clearly communicate** expectations for learning and behavior that are developmentally appropriate and applied equitably. Describe the goals of the lesson and relate them to your students' lives and the real world.
- **Ensure** lessons are linked to standards and that student learning is sequential and builds upon prior lessons.
- **Be flexible** with instructional strategies to allow for teachable moments and personalization of lessons.
- **Use** student-centered pedagogy and appropriate classroom management and discipline strategies that meet students' diverse needs and learning styles.

- **Engage** students in appropriate leadership positions and decision-making processes in the classroom and school.
- **Establish** a reward system for both academic and extracurricular achievements, but also encourage the intrinsic rewards of learning and excelling in extracurricular programs.
- **Fairly** enforce reasonable and consistent disciplinary policies.
- **Encourage** open, respectful communication about differing viewpoints.
- **Advocate** for class-size reduction to ensure more time for individualized assistance.

Participate in Professional Development Opportunities to Enhance Your Abilities to Meet the Diverse Needs of Your Students

- **Further** develop your expertise in child and adolescent development, and share lessons learned with other school staff to increase understanding about the needs of the students.
- **Participate** in professional development opportunities on implementing required school curricula, using effective teaching methods, and organizing the classroom and school to promote a positive environment.
- **Attend** workshops and trainings on communicating effectively with and involving parents in school activities, and share ideas for involving parents with other staff at your school.
- **Request** materials, time, resources, and support to use the skills you learn in training.
- **Form** learning teams to observe experienced teachers who effectively manage classrooms and facilitate group work.
- **Coach or mentor** other teachers and staff to develop effective teaching techniques and classroom management strategies, and engage in creative problem-solving.

Promote Open Communication, Trust, and Caring among School Staff, Families, and Community Partners

- **Communicate** expectations, values, and norms that support positive health and academic behaviors to your peers throughout the school community.
- **Provide** opportunities for students of all levels to interact, develop friendships, and engage in teamwork.
- **Support** student clubs and activities that promote a positive school climate, such as gay-straight alliances and multicultural clubs.
- **Create** opportunities such as, internships and service-learning projects for students to partner with and help adults.
- **Commit** to and model respectful behavior toward principals, other teachers, and school staff.

- **Challenge** all school staff to greet each student by name.
- **Encourage** teachers, counselors, health service professionals, coaches, and other school staff to build stronger relationships with students who are experiencing academic or personal issues.
- **Request** access to a school counselor, psychologist, or other expert for consultations or student referrals when needed.

School Connectedness Is Especially Important for At-Risk Youth

School connectedness is particularly important for young people who are at increased risk for feeling alienated or isolated from others. Any student who is "different" from the social norm may have difficulty connecting with other students and adults in the school, and may be more likely to feel unsafe. Those at greater risk for feeling disconnected include students with disabilities, students who are lesbian, gay, bisexual, transgender, or question their sexual orientation, students who are homeless, or any student who is chronically truant due to a variety of circumstances. Strong family involvement and supportive school personnel, inclusive school environments, and curricula that reflect the realities of a diverse student body can help students become more connected to their school.

CHAPTER 37

POSITIVE YOUTH DEVELOPMENT FOR SEXUAL MINORITIES

About This Chapter: Text in this chapter begins with excerpts from "LGBT Youth," Centers for Disease Control and Prevention (CDC), June 21, 2017; Text beginning with the heading "Parents' Influence on the Health of Lesbian, Gay, and Bisexual Teens: What Parents and Families Should Know" is excerpted from "Parents' Influence on the Health of Lesbian, Gay, and Bisexual Teens: What Parents and Families Should Know," Centers for Disease Control and Prevention (CDC), November 2013. Reviewed August 2020.

Most lesbian, gay, bisexual (LGB) youth are happy and thrive during their adolescent years. Having a school that creates a safe and supportive learning environment for all students and having caring and accepting parents are especially important. Positive environments can help all youth achieve good grades and maintain good mental and physical health. However, some LGB youth are more likely than their heterosexual peers to experience negative health and life outcomes.

For youth to thrive in schools and communities, they need to feel socially, emotionally, and physically safe and supported. A positive school climate has been associated with decreased depression, suicidal feelings, substance use, and unexcused school absences among LGB students.

What Schools Can Do

Schools can implement evidence-based policies, procedures, and activities designed to promote a healthy environment for all youth, including LGB students. For example, research has shown that in schools with LGB support groups (such as gay-straight alliances), LGB students were less likely to experience threats of violence, miss school because they felt unsafe, or attempt suicide than those students in schools without LGB support groups. A recent study found that LGB students had fewer suicidal thoughts and attempts when schools had gay-straight alliances and policies prohibiting expression of homophobia in place for 3 or more years.

To help promote health and safety among LGB youth, schools can implement the following policies and practices:

- Encourage respect for all students and prohibit bullying, harassment, and violence against all students.
- Identify "safe spaces," such as counselors' offices or designated classrooms, where LGB youth can receive support from administrators, teachers, or other school staff.
- Encourage student-led and student-organized school clubs that promote a safe, welcoming, and accepting school environment (e.g., gay-straight alliances or gender and sexuality alliances, which are school clubs open to youth of all sexual orientations and genders).
- Ensure that health curricula or educational materials include human immunodeficiency virus (HIV), other STD, and pregnancy prevention information that is relevant to LGB youth (such as ensuring that curricula or materials use language and terminology).
- Provide training to school staff on how to create safe and supportive school environments for all students, regardless of sexual orientation or gender identity, and encourage staff to attend these training sessions.
- Facilitate access to community-based providers who have experience providing health services, including HIV/STD testing and counseling, social, and psychological services to lesbian, gay, bisexual, transgender, and queer/questioning (LGBTQ) youth.

Parents' Influence on the Health of Lesbian, Gay, and Bisexual Teens: What Parents and Families Should Know

The teen years can be a challenging time for young people and their parents. This chapter provides information on how parents can promote positive health outcomes for their lesbian, gay, or bisexual (LGB) teen. The information is based on a review of published studies, which found that parents play an important role in shaping the health of their LGB teen.

When LGB teens share their sexual orientation (or even if they choose not to share it), they may feel rejected by important people in their lives, including their parents. This rejection can negatively influence an LGB teen's overall well-being.

On the other hand, a positive family environment, with high levels of parental support and low levels of conflict, is associated with LGB youth who experience healthy emotional adjustment. These teens are less likely to engage in sexual risk behaviors and be involved in violence.

How Parents Make a Difference

Research suggests that LGB teens experience better health outcomes when their parents support their sexual orientation in positive and affirming ways. Compared to

> Compared to heterosexual youth, LGB teens are more likely to experience bullying, physical violence, or rejection. As a result, LGB teens are at an increased risk for suicidal thoughts and behaviors and report higher rates of sexual risk behavior and substance abuse.

teens who do not feel valued by their parents, LGB youth who feel valued by their parents are less likely to:

- Experience depression
- Attempt suicide
- Use drugs and alcohol
- Become infected with sexually transmitted diseases

Specific Actions for Parents

Research on parenting shows how important it is—regardless of their teen's sexual orientation—for parents to:

- Have open, honest conversations with their teens about sex
- Know their teen's friends and know what their teen is doing
- Develop common goals with their teen, including being healthy and doing well in school

Although additional research is needed to better understand the associations between parenting and the health of LGB youth, the following are research-based action steps parents can take to support the health and well-being of their LGB teen and decrease the chances that their teen will engage in risky behaviors.

Talk and Listen

- Parents who talk with and listen to their teen in a way that invites an open discussion about sexual orientation can help their teen feel loved and supported.
- When their teen is ready, parents can brainstorm her or him on how to talk with others about the teen's sexual orientation.
- Parents can talk with their teen about how to avoid risky behavior and unsafe or high-risk situations.
- Parents can talk with their teen about the consequences of bullying. Parents (and their teen) should report any physical or verbal abuse that occurs at school to teachers and the school principal.

Provide Support

- Parents need to understand that teens find it very stressful to share their sexual orientation.

- Parents who take time to come to terms with how they feel about their teen's sexual orientation will be more able to respond calmly and use respectful language.
- Parents should discuss with their teen how to practice safe, healthy behaviors.

Stay Involved

- By continuing to include their teen in family events and activities, parents can help their teen feel supported.
- Parents can help their teen develop a plan for dealing with challenges, staying safe, and reducing risk.
- Parents who make an effort to know their teen's friends and romantic partners and know what their teen is doing can help their teen stay safe and feel cared about.

Be Proactive

- Parents who build positive relationships with their teen's teachers and school personnel can help ensure a safe and welcoming learning environment.
- If parents think their teen is depressed or needs other mental-health support, they should speak with a school counselor, social worker, psychologist, or other health professional.
- Parents can access many organizations and online information resources to learn more about how they can support their LGB teen, other family members, and their teen's friends.
- Parents can help their teen find appropriate LGB organizations and go with their teen to events and activities that support LGB youth.

CHAPTER 38
DEALING WITH BULLYING

About This Chapter: Text in this chapter begins with excerpts from "What Teens Can Do," StopBullying. gov, U.S. Department of Health and Human Services (HHS), February 7, 2018; Text beginning with the heading "Report Cyberbullying" is excerpted from "Report Cyberbullying," StopBullying.gov, U.S. Department of Health and Human Services (HHS), February 8, 2018.

Bullying stops us from being who we want to be, and prevents us from expressing ourselves freely, and might even make us feel unsafe. If you are bullied, say something! If you are bullying, it is not cool!

You Might Be Being Bullied

- **Speak up.** If you feel uncomfortable with the comments or actions of someone... tell someone! It is better to let a trusted adult know, than to let the problem continue.

What Is Bullying?

Bullying is unwanted, aggressive behavior among school-aged children that involves a real or perceived power imbalance. The behavior is repeated, or has the potential to be repeated, over time. Both kids who are bullied and who bully others may have serious, lasting problems.

In order to be considered bullying, the behavior must be aggressive and include:

- **An imbalance of power.** Kids who bully use their power—such as physical strength, access to embarrassing information, or popularity—to control or harm others. Power imbalances can change over time and in different situations, even if they involve the same people.
- **Repetition.** Bullying behaviors happen more than once or have the potential to happen more than once.

Bullying includes actions such as making threats, spreading rumors, attacking someone physically or verbally, and excluding someone from a group on purpose.

(Source: "What Is Bullying," StopBullying.gov, U.S. Department of Health and Human Services (HHS))

- **Get familiar with what bullying is and what it is not.** If you recognize any of the descriptions, you should stay calm, stay respectful, and tell an adult as soon as possible.

   If you feel like you are at risk of harming yourself or others get help now!

Someone Is Bullying You Online or via Text Message
- Remember, bullying does not only happen at school. It can happen anywhere, including through texting, the Internet, and social media.

You Do Not Get Bullied, but Your Friend Does
Stop Bullying on the Spot
When adults respond quickly and consistently to bullying behavior they send the message that it is not acceptable. Research shows this can stop bullying behavior over time. There are simple steps adults can take to stop bullying on the spot and keep kids safe.

Do's
- Intervene immediately. It is ok to get another adult to help.
- Separate the kids involved.
- Make sure everyone is safe.
- Meet any immediate medical or mental-health needs.
- Stay calm. Reassure the kids involved, including bystanders.
- Model respectful behavior when you intervene.

Avoid These Common Mistakes
- Do not ignore it. Do not think kids can work it out without adult help.
- Do not immediately try to sort out the facts.
- Do not force other kids to say publicly what they saw.
- Do not question the children involved in front of other kids.
- Do not talk to the kids involved together, only separately.
- Do not make the kids involved apologize or patch up relations on the spot.

   Get police help or medical attention immediately if:
   - A weapon is involved
   - There are threats of serious physical injury
   - There are threats of hate-motivated violence, such as racism or homophobia
   - There is serious bodily harm
   - There is sexual abuse

   Anyone is accused of an illegal act, such as robbery or extortion—using force to get money, property, or services.

You Want to Contribute to Antibullying Initiatives in Your School or Community

The Federal Partners in Bullying Prevention invite you to take action to make a difference in your community! You can join other youth leaders across the country and the Federal Partners to organize a bullying prevention social and educational event.

Report Cyberbullying

When cyberbullying happens, it is important to document and report the behavior so it can be addressed.

Steps to Take Immediately

- Do not respond to and do not forward cyberbullying messages.
- Keep evidence of cyberbullying. Record the dates, times, and descriptions of instances when cyberbullying has occurred. Save and print screenshots, emails, and text messages. Use this evidence to report cyberbullying to web and cell phone service providers.
- Block the person who is cyberbullying.

Report Cyberbullying to Online Service Providers

Cyberbullying often violates the terms of service established by social media sites and Internet service providers (ISPs).

- Review their terms and conditions or rights and responsibilities sections. These describe content that is or is not appropriate.
- Visit social media safety centers to learn how to block users and change settings to control who can contact you.
- Report cyberbullying to the social media site so they can take action against users abusing the terms of service.

Report Cyberbullying to Law Enforcement

When cyberbullying involves these activities it is considered a crime and should be reported to law enforcement:

- Threats of violence
- Child pornography or sending sexually explicit messages or photos
- Taking a photo or video of someone in a place where she or he would expect privacy
- Stalking and hate crimes

Some states consider other forms of cyberbullying criminal. Consult your state's laws and law enforcement for additional guidance.

Report Cyberbullying to Schools

- Cyberbullying can create a disruptive environment at school and is often related to in-person bullying. The school can use the information to help inform prevention and response strategies.
- In many states, schools are required to address cyberbullying in their antibullying policy. Some state laws also cover off-campus behavior that creates a hostile school environment.

CHAPTER 39
LEARNING TO RESIST PEER PRESSURE

About This Chapter: Text beginning with the heading "Peer Pressure" is excerpted from "Peer Pressure," Office of Adolescent Health (OAH), U.S. Department of Health and Human Services (HHS), March 25, 2019; Text beginning with the heading "Resisting Peer Pressure" is excerpted from "Resisting Peer Pressure," National Institute on Drug Abuse (NIDA) for Teens, August 14, 2017.

Peer Pressure

Friends can influence an adolescent's attitudes and behaviors in ways that matter across multiple domains of health and well-being, well into adulthood. We often hear about this in the form of peer pressure, which refers more explicitly to the pressure adolescents feel from their friends or peer group to behave in certain ways, good or bad. It can take the form of encouragement, requests, challenges, threats, or insults. Sometimes, peer pressure is unspoken—an adolescent may feel pressured to do something simply because their friends are doing it.

Research shows that friends and peer groups are linked to adolescents' positive and negative:

- Health behaviors, including their diet and level of physical activity;
- Risk behaviors, including tobacco use, marijuana use, alcohol use, and use of other drugs;
- School engagement, including their grade point average (GPA) and attitudes towards school;
- Tastes in clothing and entertainment; and
- Dating behaviors and formation of sexual identities and romantic partnerships.

Emerging research indicates that social acceptance by peers triggers stronger positive emotions during adolescence than it does in adulthood, which may be one reason youth are so keen to fit in. Additionally, teens, unlike adults, are more likely to ignore risks in favor of rewards when making a decision.

Talking with Teens about Peer Relationships

Friends are really important to teens. And as teens grow, parents recognize that friends play bigger and bigger roles in their lives. They become romantic partners. They help teens develop social skills, try new activities, and provide them with lots of support and encouragement. Through their friends, teens figure out a lot about themselves and who they are becoming. Teens who have trouble forming positive friendship relationships can struggle in many areas of their life.

On the other hand, parents often worry that teens' friends are not always good influences. They may isolate, tease, or bully each other. They may promote attitudes and behaviors that parents do not like. And they can put a lot of pressure on each other to be sexually active; use alcohol, tobacco, and other drugs; and engage in other risky behaviors.

Even though parents cannot control teen relationships, they have a lot of influence on their teens' friendship choices and the quality of those relationships, including romantic relationships. Through both your modeling and your actions, you can guide your teens toward the kinds of positive peer relationships that help them make better choices and grow up successfully.

(Source: "Talking with Teens about Peer Relationships," Office of Adolescent Health (OAH), U.S. Department of Health and Human Services (HHS)

Generally, young adolescents are the most susceptible to peer pressure, and recent research indicates that popular adolescents may be under higher pressure than other youth to conform to peer behaviors. While popular adolescents often possess a wider range of social skills and better knowledge about themselves than other youth, popularity can be associated with higher rates of alcohol and substance use, vandalism, and shoplifting.

Adolescent Friendship Difficulties

Healthy friendships matter across the life course. Examining the lifelong health benefits from friendships in adolescence is an emerging field of research. There is some evidence that healthy adolescent friendships contribute to healthy long-term outcomes, such as physical activity. Furthermore, difficulties forming healthy friendships in early adolescence can lead to trouble forming healthy friendships in late adolescence and adulthood. There are numerous difficulties adolescents can encounter in the process of making, keeping, and deepening friendships.

- Some adolescents have difficulty making friends or feel more comfortable alone. Struggling to make friends is not unusual, and parents and other caring adults can help adolescents build the skills needed to make friends. Additionally, alone time is important to adolescents. However, if adolescents spend most of their time alone and have other warning signs like difficulty sleeping, they may need mental-health support.

- Families are the first social relationships children form. Adolescents who were raised in families with limited emotional closeness or strained relationships may have difficulty with intimacy. These youths may struggle to express themselves openly and form close bonds.
- Some adolescents experience, witness, or engage in bullying, which involves repeated aggression and an imbalance of power among youth. Being bullied is linked to a range of negative outcomes, including depression, anxiety, and decreased academic achievement.
- Technology can be a challenging factor in some adolescent friendships. Conflicts between friends can originate online. While many youth use technologies to make and stay in touch with friends, others use social media and other online platforms to engage in cyberbullying. Additionally, spending more than two hours a day on sedentary screen time can be a risk factor for obesity and other health problems.
- Youth with disabilities may have additional challenges forming friendships and participating in activities.

Resisting Peer Pressure

A lot of people are standing up for what they believe in these days. Sooner or later, you will probably have the chance to do that, too. If you feel pressured into using drugs or anything else you do not want to do, you can resist.

The Power to Resist

"Resist" means you do not give in to, or go along with, something that somebody wants you to do. Resisting peer pressure can be a challenge—especially for teens, who often want to impress their friends, even if it means taking a risk.

But you can resist peer pressure with practice and a few tips.

Resistance Tips

First of all, you can remind yourself that most teens do not use alcohol or drugs.

The National Institute on Alcohol Abuse and Alcoholism (NIAAA), offers these tips for resisting an offer to use drugs or alcohol:
- Look the person in the eye.
- Speak in a polite, but clear and firm, voice.
- Suggest something else to do.
- Walk away from the situation.
- Find something else to do with other friends.

You can always blame your resistance on your parents. Say, "I'd be in big trouble if they ever found out."

Six Tactful Tips for Resisting Peer Pressure to Use Drugs and Alcohol

Even when you are confident in your decision not to use drugs or alcohol, it can be hard when it is your friend who is offering.

A lot of times, a simple "no thanks" may be enough. But sometimes it is not. It can get intense, especially if the people who want you to join in on a bad idea feel judged.

Here are a few tips that may come in handy.

1. Offer to be the designated driver. Get your friends home safely, and everyone will be glad you did not drink or take drugs.
2. If you are on a sports team, you can say you are staying healthy to maximize your athletic performance—besides, no one would argue that a hangover would help you play your best.
3. "I have to [study for a big test / go to a concert / visit my grandmother / babysit / march in a parade, etc.]. I cannot do that after a night of drinking/drugs."
4. Keep a bottled drink like a soda or iced tea with you to drink at parties. People will be less likely to pressure you to drink alcohol if you are already drinking something. If they still offer you something, just say, "I'm covered."
5. Find something to do so that you look busy. Get up and dance. Offer to DJ.
6. When all else fails...blame your parents. They won't mind! Explain that your parents are really strict, or that they will checkup on you when you get home.

(Source: "6 Tactful Tips for Resisting Peer Pressure to Use Drugs and Alcohol," National Institute on Drug Abuse (NIDA) for Teens)

CHAPTER 40
HEALTHY WAYS TO COPE WITH STRESS

About This Chapter: This chapter includes text excerpted from "Tips for Coping with Stress," Centers for Disease Control and Prevention (CDC), September 3, 2019.

Everyone—adults, teens, and even children, experiences stress. Stress is a reaction to a situation where a person feels threatened or anxious. Stress can be positive (e.g., preparing for a wedding) or negative (e.g., dealing with a natural disaster). Learning healthy ways to cope and getting the right care and support can help reduce stressful feelings and symptoms.

After a traumatic event, people may have strong and lingering reactions. These events may include personal or environmental disasters, or threats with an assault. The symptoms may be physical or emotional. Common reactions to a stressful event can include:

- Disbelief, shock, and numbness
- Feeling sad, frustrated, and helpless
- Difficulty concentrating and making decisions
- Headaches, back pains, and stomach problems
- Smoking or use of alcohol or drugs

Coping with Stress

Feeling emotional and nervous or having trouble sleeping and eating can all be normal reactions to stress. Here are some healthy ways you can deal with stress:

- **Take care of yourself.**
  - Eat healthy, well-balanced meals.
  - Exercise on a regular basis.
  - Get plenty of sleep.
  - Give yourself a break if you feel stressed out.
- **Talk to others.** Share your problems and how you are feeling and coping with a parent, friend, counselor, doctor, or pastor.

- **Avoid drugs and alcohol.** These may seem to help, but they can create additional problems and increase the stress you are already feeling.
- **Take a break.** If news events are causing your stress, take a break from listening or watching the news.
- **Recognize when you need more help.** If problems continue or you are thinking about suicide, talk to a psychologist, social worker, or professional counselor.

Tips for Parents

It is natural for children to worry when scary or stressful events happen in their lives. Talking to your children about these events can help put frightening information into a more balanced setting. Monitor what children see and hear about stressful events happening in their lives. Here are some suggestions to help children cope:

- **Maintain a normal routine.** Helping children wake up, go to sleep, and eat meals at regular times provide them a sense of stability. Going to school and participating in typical after-school activities also provide stability and extra support.
- **Talk, listen, and encourage expression.** Create opportunities for your children to talk, but do not force them. Listen to your child's thoughts and feelings and share some of yours. After a traumatic event, it is important for children to feel they can share their feelings and that you understand their fears and worries. Keep having these conversations. Ask them regularly how they feel in a week, in a month, and so on.
- **Watch and listen.** Be alert for any change in behavior. Are children sleeping more or less? Are they withdrawing from friends or family? Any changes in behavior may be signs that your child is having trouble and may need support.
- **Reassure.** Stressful events can challenge a child's sense of safety and security. Reassure your child about her or his safety and well-being. Discuss ways that you, the school, and the community are taking steps to keep them safe.
- **Connect with others.** Talk to other parents and your child's teachers about ways to help your child cope. It is often helpful for parents, schools, and health professionals to work together for the well-being of all children in stressful times.

Tips for Kids and Teens

After a traumatic event, it is normal to feel anxious about your safety and security. Even if you were not directly involved, you may worry about whether this type of event may someday affect you. Check out the tips below for some ideas to help deal with these fears.

- Talk to and stay connected to others. This might be:
  - Parents, or other relatives
  - Friends
  - Teachers
  - Coach
  - Family doctor
  - Member of your place of worship

Talking with someone can help you make sense out of your experience and figure out ways to feel better. If you are not sure where to turn, call your local crisis intervention center or a national hotline.

- **Get active.** Go for a walk, play sports, play a musical instrument, or join an after-school program. Volunteer with a community group that promotes nonviolence or another school or community activity that you care about. These can be positive ways to handle your feelings and to see that things are going to get better.
- **Take care of yourself.** Try to get plenty of sleep, eat right, exercise, and keep a normal routine. By keeping yourself healthy, you will be better able to handle a tough time.
- **Take information breaks.** Pictures and stories about a disaster can increase worry and other stressful feelings. Taking breaks from the news, Internet, and conversations about the disaster can help calm you down.

Tips for School Personnel

School personnel can help their students restore their sense of safety by talking with the children about their fears. Other tips for school personnel include:

- **Reach out and talk.** Create opportunities to have students talk, but do not force them. Try asking questions like, what do you think about these events, or how do you think these things happen? You can be a model by sharing some of your own thoughts as well as correct misinformation. When children talk about their feelings, it can help them cope and to know that different feelings are normal.
- **Watch and listen.** Be alert for any change in behavior. Are students withdrawing from friends? Acting out? These changes may be early signs that a student is struggling and needs extra support from the school and family.
- **Maintain normal routines.** A regular classroom and school schedule can provide a sense of stability and safety. Encourage students to keep up with their schoolwork and extracurricular activities but do not push them if they seem overwhelmed.

- **Take care of yourself.** You are better able to support your students if you are healthy, coping and taking care of yourself first.
  - Eat healthy, well-balanced meals.
  - Exercise on a regular basis.
  - Get plenty of sleep.
  - Give yourself a break if you feel stressed out.

CHAPTER 41
HANDLING SUICIDAL THOUGHTS

Deciding to end one's own life is a result of unbearable and immeasurable distress that goes against every human instinct. Suicide may seem like the only way to find relief when life does not seem worth living anymore. It may seem as though there are no options left when a person starts to feel this way.

Symptoms of Suicidal Thoughts
Suicidal thoughts or suicide warning signs include:
- Talking about suicide and death often
- Wanting to break from social interaction and stay isolated
- Having extreme mood swings
- Being severely agitated
- Feeling trapped or hopeless
- Irregular sleeping and eating patterns
- Excessive use of alcohol or drugs
- Self-destructive behavior, such as drug usage or reckless driving
- Looking out for lethal means, such as purchasing a gun or stockpiling pills
- Sudden personality changes

A few things to remember whenever you feel emotionally low are:
- Ending your life is not the only way to get out of your problems.
- Your problems are not going to be permanent. Things will change and things will get better with time.
- There are still so many things left for you to achieve in life.
- Emotions are not going to be the same. They keep changing constantly. What is felt today may not be same tomorrow.
- Your death will create grief and anguish in the lives of your loved ones.

Feeling suicidal or having suicidal thoughts is not a defect in the character. Many people have/had such thoughts at some point in their lives. Having such feelings and thoughts does not mean a person is crazy, weak, or flawed. It is easy for a person undergoing suicidal thoughts to overcome such pain and problems with time and the support of people.

Adequate Steps to Prevent Suicide

The measurable steps that are to be taken while feeling suicidal are:

Avoid Hasty Decisions

Hasty decisions and actions should not be made when you are in a depressed state of mind. It is good to restrain oneself from such thoughts for at least 24 hours.

Avoid Drugs and Alcohol

Drugs and alcohol can induce suicidal thoughts. Nonprescription drugs or alcohol should be avoided when feeling hopeless.

Make Your Home Safe

Hurtful things such as pills, knives, razors, and firearms should be removed from homes. An overdose of medications should also be avoided.

Do Not Keep These Suicidal Feelings to Yourself

It is clearly understood that sharing our feelings, emotions, and sadness is the first step to coping with suicidal thoughts. It can be to a friend, family member, therapist, teacher, coach, counselor, or anyone whom you trust. Find a person who can be trusted and let them know how bad things are. Fear, shame, or embarrassment should not prevent you from seeking help. Do not let anxiety, guilt or humiliation stop you from searching for support.

Open Up

Talking with trusted friends and acquaintances face to face, and spending time with them is very helpful to avoid negative thoughts.

Stick to a Schedule

Make a written schedule and stick to it every day, no matter what. A regular routine helps to control emotions.

Move Out of the Cocoon

Stepping out of home or into nature for at least 30 minutes a day helps to calm the mind.

Involve in Physical Activities

Exercising and physical activity boosts the mind and morale. A minimum of 30 minutes of exercise every day brings a positive effect on the mood.

Remember Your Personal Goals

Traveling to a particular place, reading a specific book, owning a pet, moving to another place, learning a new hobby, volunteering, and making time to do things that bring joy to you are a few goals that help to ease the mind.

Things to Avoid Suicidal Tendencies

- **Solitude.** Solitude can intensify suicidal thoughts. Always be with someone you love or trust. Pick up the phone to dial a helpline during a crisis.
- **Things that make you feel worse.** Hearing sad songs, searching for photographs, reading old documents, or visiting the grave of a loved one will all contribute to the bad feelings. Avoid alcohol and drugs as they can have a psychological impact and worsen your mood. Also stay away from negative thoughts.
- Admitting suicidal thoughts to another person even though you trust them can be difficult.
- Talk to that person you trust and share with her/him what exactly is being felt. It has to be clearly mentioned if you have suicidal tendencies.
- If it is too difficult for you to talk about your feelings, try writing it down in a note and handing it to the person you trust.

What If You Do Not Feel Understood

If it appears like the first person you reached out to does not understand, inform someone else or dial a helpline for a suicidal crisis. Allow no negative experience to discourage you from seeking anyone's support.

Suicide Crisis Lines in the United States

- National Suicide Prevention Lifeline at 800-273-8255 or IMAlive at 800-784-2433
- The Trevor Project offers suicide prevention services for LGBTQ youth at 866-488-7386.
- SAMHSA's National Helpline offers referrals for substance abuse and mental-health treatment at 800-662-4357.

References

1. Jaffe, Jaelline; Robinson, Lawrence; Segal, Jeanne. "Are You Feeling Suicidal?" Help guide, April 16, 2020.
2. "Suicide and Suicidal Thoughts," Mayo Foundation for Medical Education and Research (MFMER), October 18, 2018.

CHAPTER 42

INCREASING MENTAL-HEALTH LITERACY, HELP-SEEKING ATTITUDES, AND REDUCING STIGMA

About This Chapter: Text in this chapter begins with excerpts from "Peer Programs: A Solution for Youth by Youth Samskruthi—California," National Institute on Minority Health and Health Disparities (NIMHD), September 25, 2019; Text under the heading "Mental-Health Literacy" is excerpted from "Vitalis Jasmine—Colorado," National Institute on Minority Health and Health Disparities (NIMHD), September 25, 2019; Text under the heading "Help-Seeking Attitude and Reducing Stigma" is excerpted from "Breaching the Stigma: Improving Mental Health Education Amanda—Maryland," National Institute on Minority Health and Health Disparities (NIMHD), September 25, 2019; Text under the heading "Attitudes and Discrimination" is excerpted from "Attitudes and Discrimination," Youth.gov, November 1, 2012. Reviewed August 2020.

Though 50 percent of mental illnesses appear by the age of 14, the average lag between onset and getting help is 8 to 10 years. Due to issues such as stigma, lack of accessibility, and lack of inclusivity in mental-healthcare systems, adolescents often do not receive the help they need until there is a crisis. The most effective way to bring help to youth is through peer programs, which reduce stigma, increase mental-health literacy, and encourage students to get the most effective and comfortable help available for them.

A large barrier facing youth who struggle with mental health is stigma due to a lack of mental-health education. Mental health is often viewed as taboo, resulting in the toxic mindset that mental illness is weak and abnormal. Stigma makes it difficult for youth to understand and cope with their mental-health issues, while also making them feel alone in their struggle. This loneliness is furthered by the fact that youth are often unable to discuss their mental health with peers or with parents.

Data from the Born This Way Foundation affirms that 49 percent of youth rarely or never talk about their mental health, despite 88 percent of youth acknowledging mental health as a priority. Adding to this suffocating burden, teens with mental-health issues are forced to reach out for help on their own with little guidance. According to the Born This Way Foundation, 47 percent of youth cite not knowing where to go for help as their key barrier to receiving mental-health services. Stigma at all steps on the journey to help, from difficulty recognizing mental-health issues to the lack of guidance in seeking services, bars youth from getting help.

However, even when youth make the decision to seek help, they face a new set of difficulties in mental-healthcare systems, which are often inaccessible. For example, 42 percent of youth cite their inability to afford mental healthcare as their main barrier to getting help. Mental-health services are often too expensive for youth to pay, excluding low-income youth as well as youth whose parents or guardians are unwilling to support their decision.

In addition, mental healthcare is often less accessible to youth of ethnic minorities. Of African American and Native American youth, 40 percent and 48 percent respectively reported that their communities rarely or never have access to youth mental-health resources, as opposed to 28 percent of white youth. This reflects the lack of cultural competence in youth mental-healthcare systems, which leaves whole subsets of the population whose struggles are not understood. Another systemic issue is the focus on pathologization in mental-healthcare systems. This approach is harmful because it does not account for the environmental and social factors that contribute to mental health, which may not necessarily be tied to a diagnosable illness. In addition, since mental-health services are most often found in clinical settings that focus on treatment rather than building trust and comfort, youth who are surrounded by stigma often feel uncomfortable seeking out this kind of help. Current mental-health services fail to account for the unique challenges and diverse experiences that contribute to youth mental health. The challenge for mental-health systems, therefore, is to reach youth in a more effective way that reaches past stigma to people of all experiences.

School-Based Peer Support Programs

A solution is to invest in the implementation of peer programs in all school districts. Peer programs are groups of student leaders who are trained to increase mental-health literacy and discussion. While they do not necessarily provide counseling themselves, peer programs are incredibly effective in reducing stigma and encouraging students to seek appropriate help. Youth in peer programs often initiate a variety of mental-health projects within their schools that incorporate discussions and activities that encourage youth to understand and discuss mental health. This has proven effective in Michigan, where implementing a peer program saw a significant reduction in stigma and a significant increase in people willing to talk to their peers about mental health.

In addition, since youth have an understanding of the unique challenges faced by their student body, they are able to create effective change. As peer leaders interact with others, they are able to support those struggling with mental-health issues and guide them toward the best options for their treatment. This is facilitated both by the reduction of stigma and by the trustworthy environment created by peer leaders. With their diverse lived experiences, training, and knowledge of the school community, these youth could guide others to the most effective and comfortable service for them. This guidance is crucial, especially since youth often have to navigate the world of treatment on their own. In Michigan, youth in schools with peer programs reported a higher likelihood of seeking professional help and knowing where to go. Therefore, peer programs are a unique way to bring comfortable guidance and long-term reduction of stigma directly to youth communities.

Another facet of peer programs could be the development of support groups with peer leaders as facilitators who can guide the group to resources. Involving youth with a variety of identities and lived experiences in peer programs is crucial to maximizing success. Forming groups of youth with similar struggles ignites trust and a connection that makes students feel heard and more comfortable seeking help. In addition, they could help youth who do not have access to services due to a lack of familial support, since support groups would be held at school for no cost. They also serve as a vehicle for youth to talk about their mental health with people they trust, which removes the discomfort that often accompanies clinical services. This is especially useful in groups that often have less access to mental-health services, such as Asian youth, African-American youth, Native-American youth, foster youth, and LGBTQ+ youth. In support groups, the peer leaders could also share the resources that would be best suited to their group based on personal experience and training, eliminating the barrier of youth not knowing where to go.

Mental-Health Literacy

To build mental-health literacy, students should be required to take a health class that discusses the intricacies of mental health for more than a week, treats mental health like physical health, and emphasizes that others also have mental illnesses.

Even then, every second matters, and current society is lagging behind. Given that suicide is one of the leading causes of adolescent death, proactive schools can offer the primary introduction to mental health, but individual protocols must ensue. Just as having an annual physical, just as going to the dentist, meeting a psychiatrist and having an annual mental-health checkup should be the norm. Since currently 70 percent of a Primary Care Physician's (PCP) practice involves psychological issues, mental-health needs to be integrated into primary care. Still, no PCP can replace a psychiatrist, so these professions must be encouraged so that professional help is no longer too expensive or too far away. Finding and receiving help cannot be the fight.

Colie's Closet—a peer education group aiming to educate and remove the stigma around mental health. Colie's has set a successful precedent in the United States for promoting peer mental-health education. It targets the problem of limited knowledge and awareness regarding mental health, which ultimately is the root of the stigma that keeps growing. Teachers need to be knowledgeable about depression, suicide, risk factors, warning signs, and steps to take when concerned about a student. Support is available through free eLearning courses on Alison or even a $20 Mental Health First Aid Course. Teachers can be both a source of knowledge and a source of support. They can feel equipped to foster simple conversations in each class to address mental health while building a welcoming community. Whether this occurs once a day or even once a year, it would be such a drastic difference to what exists now. In doing so, teachers could be an integral part in breaking the stigma.

Help-Seeking Attitude and Reducing Stigma

In a country that often treats white as default and minorities as afterthoughts, minorities seem to have no choice, but to be perfect. Admitting to mental-health disorders is, unfortunately, still seen as a sign of failure. To combat this stigma, society must treat mental illnesses as seriously as it does physical illnesses.

No physical illness invites as much shame and social stigma as mental illnesses do. When a person is afflicted with the flu or breaks a bone, it is expected that she or he will receive adequate medical treatment. Misconceptions of mental health, however, lead many to believe that mental illnesses can simply be cured by cheering up or trying harder. A large part of this issue is a lack of education on the subject of mental health.

Mental illness is often seen as the victim's fault, when in reality, it is generally caused by uncontrollable chemical imbalances in the brain. Research has suggested that people who have depression, for example, have unbalanced levels of neurotransmitters such as serotonin, dopamine, and norepinephrine. Scientific progress has allowed for the development of drugs that treat patients by blocking the neurotransmitter glutamate or regulating hormone levels. To keep pace with these scientific developments, Biology and Health curriculums in schools should be updated to teach mental illnesses as they do physical illnesses, covering the scientific causes, effects, and possible treatments available.

Recognizing mental-health disorders as illnesses will both decrease the stigma against them and allow teenagers to better understand the resources available to them. Students should be taught the warning signs of depression, but they should also understand that like any health disease, mental illnesses do not always exhibit textbook symptoms.

Social media platforms often exacerbate detrimental comparisons among adolescents: since people generally post about their best moments, it can seem to each of us like we are alone in our hardships. This feeling of isolation can contribute to more shame and stigma against the topic of mental illness. However, social media does not have to be a negative force. Many famous influencers, including celebrities like J.K. Rowling and Michael Phelps, have opened up their own experiences with mental illness. Seeing successful people overcome mental illness can uplift teenagers and encourage them to seek the help they need. Public figures should continue to use their platforms to promote mental-health awareness.

Attitudes and Discrimination

Discrimination against youth with mental-health challenges begins early and increases over time, causing attitudes to become ingrained. Despite the fact that an overwhelming majority of Americans believe that people with mental illnesses are not to blame for their conditions (84%), only about 57.3 percent believe that people are generally caring and sympathetic toward individuals with mental illnesses. This percentage is much lower (24.6%) for those who themselves suffer poor mental health.

Attitudes of Young People

Discrimination and misconceptions about people with mental illnesses is prevalent for youth and young adults. Findings from a health survey suggest that, for young adults between the ages of 18 and 24:

- About 24 percent believe that a person with a mental illness is dangerous and 38.9 percent believe she or he is unpredictable.
- Less than half (44.3%) believe that someone with a mental illness can be successful at work.
- Only slightly more than half (55.2%) believe that treatment can help people with mental illnesses lead normal lives.
- Only around 26.9 percent believe that a person with mental illness can eventually recover.

Discrimination as a Barrier to Recovery

Discrimination associated with mental illness poses a large barrier to recovery and is one of the main reasons why people do not seek help and treatment. Further, an unwillingness to seek help because of the negative attitudes attached to mental health and substance abuse disorders or to suicidal thoughts has been found to be one of the risk factors associated with suicide.

What Can Be Done to Limit Discrimination?

Youth are a key population on which to focus discrimination reduction efforts, as they are more likely than the general public to know someone with a mental illness, and therefore, have a unique opportunity to make a difference. The National Annenberg Survey of Youth conducted a large scale study on these negative attitudes and found that youth who were informed with facts and able to dispel myths about individuals with mental-health disorders were less likely to discriminate against them. They concluded that various approaches have promise in decreasing negative attitudes and discrimination, such as the use of mass media to influence the attitudes of youth and educating students by incorporating persons with mental-health disorders as speakers in classroom presentations and discussions.

The Substance Abuse and Mental Health Services Administration (SAMHSA) has launched an antidiscrimination campaign called "What a Difference a Friend Makes." The premise of the campaign is that recovery from mental illness is more likely in a society that is accepting, and that provides education and support from friends. Through acceptance and social inclusion, individuals who have behavioral health challenges or mental illness can be contributing members of their families and communities.

Everyone can do something to help a person with mental illness by:

- Avoiding the use of negative labels
- Showing kindness and respect
- Helping to eliminate discrimination in housing, employment, or education

In addition, understanding and accepting friends play an important role in recovery.

- Friends can help by offering reassurance, companionship, and emotional strength.
- Friends can express an interest and concern for people with a mental illness by asking questions, listening to ideas, and being responsive.
- Friends can help encourage others to treat mental illness like any other healthcare condition.
- Friends can dismiss any preconceived notions about mental illness and embrace a more helpful way of relating to people.

PART 5 | LIVING WITH A MENTAL-HEALTH CONDITION

CHAPTER 43

HOW TO ACCESS MENTAL-HEALTH SERVICES

> About This Chapter: Text in this chapter begins with excerpts from "Access to Adolescent Mental Health Care," Office of Adolescent Health (OAH), U.S. Department of Health and Human Services (HHS), January 15, 2019; Text beginning with the heading "Where to Go for Help and Treatment" is excerpted from "A Roadmap to Behavioral Health," Centers for Medicare & Medicaid Services (CMS), August 15, 2019.

Adolescents ages 12 to 17 receive mental-health services in a variety of settings. In 2016, 3.6 million received mental-health services such as seeing a psychiatrist, psychologist, or counselor in a specialty mental-health setting, 3.2 million received services such as counseling or participating in a behavioral health program in an educational setting, and 708,000 received mental-health services from a pediatrician or family physician.

As symptoms of mental illness emerge and develop, they have strong influences on an adolescent's behavior and can become more difficult to treat. Although effective therapies exist for many mental illnesses, not all adolescents who need treatment receive it.

Where to Go for Help and Treatment

Some people find it difficult to talk about mental-health or substance-use concerns. However, this is a normal conversation to have with a healthcare provider who will respect your privacy. If you have a primary care doctor or nurse, you can start your conversation there.

There are different ways to find a doctor. People get their behavioral healthcare in many places like a primary care provider, behavioral health provider, or the emergency department (ED) or emergency room (ER) in a hospital.

Occasionally, primary care and behavioral health providers are co-located, so they are in the same building or part of the same clinic, hospital, or health center, so your care is being provided all in one place.

There are big differences between visits to your provider and visits to the emergency department like cost, time you wait for care, and follow-up.

A primary care provider is usually who you see first. The provider may offer recommended screenings. The provider will keep your health records, help you manage your ongoing health needs, and may also connect you to a behavioral health provider.

Behavioral health providers are specially trained to work with people experiencing mental and substance-use problems. They work in hospitals, community mental-health clinics, substance-use treatment centers, primary care clinics, school-based health centers, college counseling centers, and private practices.

If you have an emergency or life-threatening situation, go to the emergency department or call 911. A visit to the emergency department will cost you more than an office visit. You may wait longer at a hospital to be seen and will have fewer choices about who you see and what type of services you receive.

Finding a Behavioral Health Provider

An important step to getting behavioral healthcare is finding a provider. There are different ways to do this:

- Primary care providers (such as a doctor, nurse practitioner, or other healthcare provider) may be able to screen or treat many behavioral health problems.
- A primary care provider may also recommend or refer you to a behavioral health provider. You may need a referral for your health plan to pay for a visit. Check with your insurance company or call the behavioral health provider's office to be sure they accept your insurance and are an in-network provider.
- Sometimes insurance plans require a preauthorization. This is a decision made by the insurance plan that a service, treatment, or prescription drug is medically necessary.
- Insurance Plan Directory
- Call your insurance company or state Medicaid and Children's Health Insurance Program (CHIP), look at their website, or check your member handbook to find behavioral health providers in your network. You may want to double check to make sure the information is up-to-date.
- Use the plan directory to search for particular needs, such as a provider who speaks a language other than English, can accommodate mobility challenges, is located near you, or works with specific populations.
- Recommendations from family, friends, and other sources
- Ask family, friends, or another person in your community for a suggestion.
- Check with your insurance company or call the behavioral health provider's office to be sure they accept your insurance and are an in-network provider.

A Network is the facilities, providers, and suppliers your health insurer has an agreement with to provide you with healthcare services.

Contact your insurance company to find out which providers are "in-network." These providers may also be called "preferred-providers" or "participating providers."

If a provider is "out-of-network" it might cost you more.

Networks can change. Check with your provider each time you make an appointment.

Types of Behavioral Health Providers

There are different types of behavioral health providers. Ask your primary care provider for help deciding which provider type is right for you.

Some examples include:

- Psychiatrists diagnose mental and substance-use disorders, prescribe and monitor medications, and may provide counseling and therapy.
- Psychiatric or Mental Health Nurse Practitioners are nurses trained to provide assessment, diagnosis, and therapy for mental or substance use disorders. They can also prescribe medication. These providers may be called "Advanced Registered Nurse Practitioner" (ARNP), Advanced Practice Registered Nurse (APRN), Advanced Practice Nurse (APN), Certified Nurse Practitioner (CNP), Certified Registered Nurse Practitioner (CRNP), or Licensed Nurse Practitioner (LNP). These titles will vary depending on the state.
- Clinical psychologists make diagnoses and provide counseling and therapy. Sometimes they can prescribe medications.
- Clinical social workers make diagnoses and provide counseling and therapy, case management, and advocacy.
- Social workers provide case management and help locate treatment services and other services to support recovery and healthy living.
- Counselors make diagnoses and provide counseling. They help with improving life skills and relationships.
- Peer specialists/recovery coaches are people who have experienced mental or substance use disorders and are in recovery. They can teach you about the health system, provide emotional and social support, and help your recovery. Peers often receive training and certification.
- Substance/addiction counselors advise people who have an alcohol or other substance use disorder. They provide treatment and support to help in your recovery.

CHAPTER 44

HEALTH INSURANCE COVERAGE FOR MENTAL-HEALTH SERVICES

About This Chapter: This chapter includes text excerpted from "Recent Advances in Mental Healthcare,"
Office of Adolescent Health (OAH), U.S. Department of Health and Human Services (HHS), January 15, 2019.

The Mental Health Parity and Addiction Equity Act (MHPAEA) of 2008, the Affordable Care Act (ACA) of 2010, and the recent Medicaid expansion in many states have helped improve access to mental-health services for Americans of all ages. Parity, in health insurance plans, means that mental-health services are covered and reimbursed at the same levels as physical healthcare. Several laws address parity and equity in how health insurance plans cover mental-health services.

The Mental Health Parity Act and the Mental Health Parity and Addiction Equity Act

The Mental Health Parity Act of 1996 prohibited large group health plans from putting annual or lifetime dollar limits on mental-health benefits that are less than those put on medical/surgical benefits. The Mental Health Parity and Addiction Equity Act of 2008 added new protections, such as requiring that substance use disorders also have comparable coverage. However, MHPAEA does not require health insurance plans to include mental-health/substance-use disorders benefits; its requirements apply only to insurers that include mental-health/substance-use disorders in their existing benefit packages.

The Affordable Care Act

The Affordable Care Act of 2010 builds on the earlier parity legislation by requiring that most individual and small employer health insurance plans—including all plans offered through the health insurance Marketplace—cover mental-health and substance-use disorders services. The ACA also requires coverage of rehabilitative services that support people with behavioral health challenges. Together, these protections expand benefits for an estimated 174 million Americans. Because of the ACA, most health plans must now cover preventive services (e.g., depression screening for adults and behavioral assessments for children) at no additional cost. Most health plans cannot deny coverage, or charge more, for preexisting health conditions, including mental illnesses.

Finally, under the ACA, participants can now add or keep their children on their health insurance policy until they turn 26. Children can join or remain on a parent's plan, even if they are married, live separately from their parents, or are financially independent. In addition, those who are attending school or are eligible to enroll in their employer's plan can still be on their parent's health insurance policy. Upon turning 26, children do not have to wait for a plan's open enrollment period, but can sign up at any time.

Medicaid

All states provide some mental-health/substance-use disorders services to children who receive Medicaid. In addition, the Children's Health Insurance Program (CHIP), which works with Medicaid for eligible children, provides a variety of services including counseling, therapy, medication management, social work services, peer supports, and substance use disorder treatment. In all states, eligible children through age 18 can be covered by Medicaid and/or CHIP, and they can enroll at any time.

In addition, states can agree to a Medicaid expansion that provides coverage for eligible individuals under age 65. As of July 1, 2016, 31 states and the District of Columbia (DC) have done so. The Medicaid expansion includes benefits for people with mental-health and substance-use disorders, and coverage must meet the same parity requirements required under MHPAEA for other health plans.

CHAPTER 45
SCHOOL-BASED MENTAL-HEALTH SUPPORT

About This Chapter: Text beginning with the heading "Schools Are a Natural Setting to Support Mental Health" is excerpted from "School-Based Supports," Youth.gov, November 7, 2015. Reviewed August 2020; Text beginning with the heading "Steps for Educators to Do" is excerpted from "For Educators," MentalHealth.gov, U.S. Department of Health and Human Services (HHS), March 22, 2019.

Schools Are a Natural Setting to Support Mental Health

School-based mental health is becoming a vital part of student support systems. According to a survey, over one-third of school districts used school or district staff to provide mental-health services, and over one-fourth used outside agencies to provide mental-health services in the schools.

Mentally healthy students are more likely to go to school ready to learn, actively engage in school activities, have supportive and caring connections with adults and young people, use appropriate problem-solving skills, have nonaggressive behaviors, and add to positive school culture. Although many students are mentally healthy, the Center for Mental Health in Schools estimates that between 12 and 22 percent of school-aged children and youth have a diagnosable mental-health disorder. Because children and youth spend the majority of their time in school, schools play an increasingly critical role in supporting these students and providing a safe, nonstigmatizing, and supportive natural environment in which children, youth, and families have access to prevention, early intervention, and treatment through school-based mental-health programs.

A study by the U.S. Department of Health and Human Services (HHS) Office of Adolescent Health (OAH) indicated that adolescents are more comfortable accessing healthcare services through school-based clinics and like the idea of accessing a range of health and social services in a single location. Further, schools provide a natural setting in which students can receive needed support and services and where families are comfortable and trusting in accessing these supports and services.

Implementing School-Based Mental-Health Services

The ways school districts implement school-based mental-health services vary. They may hire school-based therapists or social workers. They can provide access to prevention programming, early identification of mental-health challenges, and treatment options. They can also partner with community mental-health organizations and agencies to develop an integrated, comprehensive program of support and services to do the following:

- Develop evidence-based programs to provide a positive school climate and promote student skills in dealing with bullying and conflicts, solving problems, developing healthy peer relationships, engaging in activities to prevent suicide and substance use, and so on.
- Develop early intervention services for students in need of additional supports such as skill groups to deal with grief, anger, anxiety, sadness, and so on.
- Develop treatment programs and services that address the various mental-health needs of students.
- Develop student and family supports and resources.
- Develop a school culture in which teachers and other student support staff are trained to recognize the early warning signs of mental-health issues with students.
- Develop a referral process to ensure that all students have equal access to services and support.

Further, early identification and referral resources may reflect a school climate that is comfortable talking about and addressing emotional health, which again may reduce the stigma often associated with receiving mental-health treatment.

Benefits of School-Based Mental-Health Services

Studies have shown the value of developing comprehensive school mental-health programs in helping students achieve academically and have access to experiences that build social skills, leadership, self-awareness, and caring connections to adults in their school and community.

Schools that also choose to collaborate with community partners have found that they can enhance the academic success of individual students. These partnerships have found to significantly improve schoolwide truancy and discipline rates, increase the rates of high school graduation, and help create a positive school environment in which a student can learn and be successful in school and in the community.

Steps for Educators to Do

Educators are often the first to notice mental-health problems. Here are some ways you can help students and their families.

What Educators Should Know

You should know:

- The warning signs for mental-health problems
- Whom to turn to, such as the principal, school nurse, school psychiatrist or psychologist, or school social worker, if you have questions or concerns about a student's behavior
- How to access crisis support and other mental-health services

What Educators Should Look For in Student Behavior

Consult with a school counselor, nurse, or administrator and the student's parents if you observe one or more of the following behaviors:

- Feeling very sad or withdrawn for more than two weeks
- Seriously trying to harm oneself, or making plans to do so
- Sudden overwhelming fear for no reason, sometimes with a racing heart or fast breathing
- Involvement in many fights or desire to badly hurt others
- Severe out-of-control behavior that can hurt oneself or others
- Not eating, throwing up, or using laxatives to make oneself lose weight
- Intense worries or fears that get in the way of daily activities
- Extreme difficulty concentrating or staying still that puts the student in physical danger or causes problems in the classroom
- Repeated use of drugs or alcohol
- Severe mood swings that cause problems in relationships
- Drastic changes in the student's behavior or personality

What Educators Can Do in Classrooms and Schools

You can support the mental health of all students in your classroom and school, not just individual students who may exhibit behavioral issues. Consider the following actions:

- Educate staff, parents, and students on symptoms of and help for mental-health problems.
- Promote social and emotional competency and build resilience.
- Help ensure a positive, safe school environment.
- Teach and reinforce positive behaviors and decision-making.
- Encourage helping others.
- Encourage good physical health.
- Help ensure access to school-based mental-health supports.

Developing Effective School Mental-Health Programs

Efforts to care for the emotional well-being of children and youth can extend beyond the classroom and into the entire school. School-based mental-health programs can focus on promoting mental wellness, preventing mental-health problems, and providing treatment.

Effective programs:

- Promote the healthy social and emotional development of all children and youth
- Recognize when young people are at risk for or are experiencing mental-health problems
- Identify how to intervene early and appropriately when there are problems

CHAPTER 46
CARING FOR YOUR MENTAL HEALTH DURING COVID-19 PANDEMIC

About This Chapter: Text beginning with the heading "Support for Teens and Young Adults" is excerpted from "Support for Teens and Young Adults," Centers for Disease Control and Prevention (CDC), July 1, 2020; Text beginning with the heading "Tips for Social Distancing, Quarantine, and Isolation during an Infectious Disease Outbreak" is excerpted from "Taking Care of Your Behavioral Health," Substance Abuse and Mental Health Services Administration (SAMHSA), January 1, 2020; Text beginning with the heading "Resources for Teens and Young Adults" is excerpted from "Resources to Support Adolescent Mental Health," Office of Adolescent Health (OAH), U.S. Department of Health and Human Services (HHS), May 3, 2017.

Support for Teens and Young Adults

Some of the questions you might be asking are, "Should I be freaking out about COVID-19?" and "Why can't I hang out with my friends in person?". You may be feeling worried, bored, or frustrated. COVID-19 is frightening, and you are not the only one feeling stressed.

While anyone can catch the virus that causes COVID-19 and people of all ages and backgrounds can get severely ill, most people have a mild illness and are able to recover at home. But regardless of your personal risk, it is natural to be concerned for your friends and family or about uncertainty and changes in your daily routine.

There are things you can do to manage your stress.
- Learn about COVID-19. Knowing the facts and stopping the spread of rumors about COVID-19 can help you feel more in control of what is happening.
- Help stop the spread of COVID-19 by washing your hands often with soap and water, covering coughs and sneezes, and avoiding close contact with other people – even your friends. COVID-19 may be spread by people who do not have symptoms. These actions will keep you from getting sick and spreading the virus to other people you care about.

- Wear masks when you do leave your home to help slow the spread of COVID-19. People who should not wear a mask are children under age 2 and anyone who has trouble breathing, or is unconscious, incapacitated, or otherwise unable to remove the mask without assistance.
- You can be social, but do it from a distance, such as reaching out to friends by phone, text, video chat, and social media.
- Find ways to relax. Take deep breaths, stretch, or meditate. Try to do activities you enjoy, like exercising, gaming, reading, or other hobbies.
- Keep to a schedule. Plan times for doing school work, relaxing, and connecting with friends.
- Avoid alcohol and drugs. These substances can weaken your body's ability to fight infections and increase the risk of certain complications associated with COVID-19.
- Talk with someone you trust about your thoughts and feelings.

You may be feeling loss or distress over the changes in your life during this time. There are steps you can take to cope with your grief.

Suicide

Different life experiences may affect the risk for suicide. For example, suicide risk is higher for those who have experienced violence, including child abuse, bullying, or sexual violence. Feelings of isolation, depression, anxiety, and other emotional or financial stresses are known to raise the risk for suicide. You may be more likely to experience these feelings during a crisis like a pandemic.

You may be particularly overwhelmed when stress is connected to a traumatic event—like a natural disaster or pandemic. Parents and educators can provide stability and support to help you feel better.

There are ways to protect against suicidal thoughts and behaviors. For example, support from family and community, or feeling connected. Reach out to others online, through social media, video chat, or by phone. Having access to in-person or virtual counseling or therapy can help with suicidal thoughts and behavior, particularly during a crisis like the COVID-19 pandemic.

Tips for Social Distancing, Quarantine, and Isolation during an Infectious Disease Outbreak

In the event of an infectious disease outbreak, local officials may require the public to take measures to limit and control the spread of the disease. The government has the right to enforce federal and state laws related to public health if people within the country get sick with highly contagious diseases that have the potential to develop into outbreaks or pandemics.

This chapter describes feelings and thoughts you may have during and after social distancing, quarantine, and isolation. It also suggests ways to care for your behavioral health during these experiences and provides resources for more help.

What to Expect: Typical Reactions
Everyone reacts differently to stressful situations such as an infectious disease outbreak that requires social distancing, quarantine, or isolation. People may feel:

Anxiety, Worry, or Fear Related To
- Your own health status
- The health status of others whom you may have exposed to the disease
- The resentment that your friends and family may feel if they need to go into quarantine as a result of contact with you
- The experience of monitoring yourself, or being monitored by others for signs and symptoms of the disease
- Time taken off from work and the potential loss of income and job security
- The challenges of securing things you need, such as groceries and personal care items
- Concern about being able to effectively care for children or others in your care
- Uncertainty or frustration about how long you will need to remain in this situation, and uncertainty about the future
- Loneliness associated with feeling cut off from the world and from loved ones
- Anger if you think you were exposed to the disease because of others' negligence

- Boredom and frustration because you may not be able to work or engage in regular day-to-day activities
- Uncertainty or ambivalence about the situation
- A desire to use alcohol or drugs to cope
- Symptoms of depression, such as feelings of hopelessness, changes in appetite, or sleeping too little or too much
- Symptoms of posttraumatic stress disorder (PTSD), such as intrusive distressing memories, flashbacks (reliving the event), nightmares, changes in thoughts and mood, and being easily startled

If you or a loved one experience any of these reactions for 2 to 4 weeks or more, contact your healthcare provider or one of the resources at the end of this chapter.

Ways to Support Yourself during Social Distancing, Quarantine, and Isolation

Understand the Risk

Consider the real risk of harm to yourself and others around you. The public perception of risk during a situation such as an infectious disease outbreak is often inaccurate. Media coverage may create the impression that people are in immediate danger when really the risk for infection may be very low. Take steps to get the facts:

- Stay up-to-date on what is happening, while limiting your media exposure. Avoid watching or listening to news reports 24/7 since this tends to increase anxiety and worry. Remember that children are especially affected by what they hear and see on television.
- Look to credible sources for information on the infectious disease outbreak.

Be Your Own Advocate

Speaking out about your needs is particularly important if you are in quarantine, since you may not be in a hospital or other facility where your basic needs are met. Ensure you have what you need to feel safe, secure, and comfortable.

- Work with local, state, or national health officials to find out how you can arrange for groceries and toiletries to be delivered to your home as needed.
- Inform healthcare providers or health authorities of any needed medications and work with them to ensure that you continue to receive those medications.

Educate Yourself

Healthcare providers and health authorities should provide information on the disease, its diagnosis, and treatment.

- Do not be afraid to ask questions—clear communication with a healthcare provider may help reduce any distress associated with social distancing, quarantine, or isolation.

- Ask for written information when available.
- Ask a family member or friend to obtain information in the event that you are unable to secure this information on your own.

Work with Your Employer to Reduce Financial Stress

If you are unable to work during this time, you may experience stress related to your job status or financial situation.

- Provide your employer with a clear explanation of why you are away from work.
- Contact the U.S. Department of Labor (DOL) toll-free at 866-487-2365 about the Family and Medical Leave Act (FMLA), which allows U.S. employees up to 12 weeks of unpaid leave for serious medical conditions, or to care for a family member with a serious medical condition.
- Contact your utility providers, cable and Internet provider, and other companies from whom you get monthly bills to explain your situation and request alternative bill payment arrangements as needed.

Connect with Others

Reaching out to people you trust is one of the best ways to reduce anxiety, depression, loneliness, and boredom during social distancing, quarantine, and isolation. You can:

- Use the telephone, email, text messaging, and social media to connect with friends, family, and others.
- Talk "face to face" with friends and loved ones using Skype or FaceTime.
- If approved by health authorities and your healthcare providers, arrange for your friends and loved ones to bring you newspapers, movies, and books.
- Sign up for emergency alerts via text or email to ensure you get updates as soon as they are available.
- Use the Internet, radio, and television to keep up with local, national, and world events.
- If you need to connect with someone because of an ongoing alcohol or drug problem, consider calling your local Alcoholics Anonymous or Narcotics Anonymous offices.

Talk to Your Doctor

If you are in a medical facility, you may have access to healthcare providers who can answer your questions. However, if you are quarantined at home, and you are worried about physical symptoms you or your loved ones may be experiencing, call your doctor or other healthcare provider.

- Ask your provider whether it would be possible to schedule remote appointments via Skype or FaceTime for mental health, substance use, or physical health needs.

- In the event that your doctor is unavailable and you are feeling stressed or are in crisis, call the hotline numbers listed at the end of this chapter for support.

Use Practical Ways to Cope and Relax

- Relax your body often by doing things that work for you—take deep breaths, stretch, meditate or pray, or engage in activities you enjoy.
- Pace yourself between stressful activities, and do something fun after a hard task.
- Talk about your experiences and feelings to loved ones and friends, if you find it helpful.
- Maintain a sense of hope and positive thinking; consider keeping a journal where you write down things you are grateful for or that are going well.

After Social Distancing, Quarantine, or Isolation

You may experience mixed emotions, including a sense of relief. If you were isolated because you had the illness, you may feel sadness or anger because friends and loved ones may have unfounded fears of contracting the disease from contact with you, even though you have been determined not to be contagious.

The best way to end this common fear is to learn about the disease and the actual risk to others. Sharing this information will often calm fears in others and allow you to reconnect with them.

If you or your loved ones experience symptoms of extreme stress—such as trouble sleeping, problems with eating too much or too little, inability to carry out routine daily activities, or using drugs or alcohol to cope—speak to a healthcare provider or call one of the hotlines below for a referral.

If you are feeling overwhelmed with emotions such as sadness, depression, anxiety, or feel like you want to harm yourself or someone else, call 911 or the National Suicide Prevention Lifeline at 800-273-TALK (800-273-8255).

Resources for Teens and Young Adults

- The Substance Abuse and Mental Health Services Administration (SAMHSA) maintains the Behavioral Health Services Locator (findtreatment.samhsa. gov), an online, map-based program that visitors can use to find facilities in their vicinity.
- SAMHSA also provides a list of suicide prevention resources for teens through its Suicide Prevention Resource Center (www.sprc.org).
- Adolescents and others experiencing suicidal crisis or emotional distress can call the National Suicide Prevention Lifeline (suicidepreventionlifeline.org) at 800-273-TALK (800-273-8255). Calls made to this 24-hour hotline are routed to the caller's nearest crisis center. People who may be uncomfortable speaking

on the phone can text the Crisis Text Line (www.crisistextline.org) at 741741 to connect with a trained crisis counselor. Texts are answered quickly 24/7.

- OK2Talk (ok2talk.org/about) is a safe, moderated online community where teens and young adults can share their stories of recovery, tragedy, struggle, or hope through creative expression such as poetry or songs, inspirational quotes, videos, and messages of support. Founding partners include the National Alliance on Mental Health (NAMI) (www.nami.org/Home), Active Minds (www.activeminds.org), and Mental Health America (MHA) (www.mhanational.org).
- NAMI's Find Support section for teens and young adults (www.nami.org/Find-Support/Teens-Young-Adults) has information on meeting with mental-health specialists, being a supportive friend, managing mental-health disorders, and more.
- The Depression and Bipolar Support Alliance (DBSA) offers local support groups (www.dbsalliance.org/support/chapters-and-support-groups) throughout the United States as well as online support groups (www.dbsalliance.org/site/PageServer?pagename=peer_Online_Support_Groups).
- College students can find support and additional resources at NAMI on Campus (www.nami.org/Get-Involved/NAMI-on-Campus) and Active Minds (www.activeminds.org)
- Office of Adolescent Health's (OAH) Adolescent Health Library provides federal resources on mental-health topics (www.hhs.gov/ash/oah/resources-and-training/adolescent-health-library/mental-health-resources-and-publications/index.html).

Resources for Youth-Serving Professionals

- **Youth Mental Health First Aid** (www.mentalhealthfirstaid.org/population-focused-modules/youth) is designed for youth and adults who regularly interact with young people. The course introduces common mental-health challenges for youth, reviews typical adolescent development, and teaches a 5-step action plan for how to help young people in both crisis and non-crisis situations. Topics covered include anxiety, depression, substance use, disorders in which psychosis may occur, disruptive behavior disorders (including AD/HD), and eating disorders.
- **NAMI Ending the Silence** (www.nami.org/Support-Education/Mental-Health-Education/NAMI-Ending-the-Silence) offers free, on-site presentations to schools and communities to teach audiences about warning signs of mental-health conditions and steps people can take if a loved one shows symptoms of mental illness. The program offers separate presentations for students, school staff, and families and includes a lead presenter and a

young adult with a mental-health condition who shares their experience of recovery.

- SAMHSA's report, Integrating Behavioral Health and Primary Care for Children and Youth: Concepts and Strategies, addresses service delivery for youth, outlines five core competencies of integrated care systems for children with behavioral health issues, and describes financing mechanisms that support integrated care systems.
- The Integrated Treatment for Co-Occurring Disorders Evidence-Based Practices (EBP) Kit (store.samhsa.gov/product/Integrated-Treatment-for-Co-Occurring-Disorders-Evidence-Based-Practices-EBP-KIT/SMA08-43660) from SAMHSA explains the principles of integrated treatment while referencing programs that successfully offer mental-health and substance-use services in one setting.
- The U.S. Department of Health and Human Services (HHS) offers mental-health resources and information at MentalHealth.gov, including guidance for educators and for community leaders.
- The Society for Adolescent Health Medicine (www.adolescenthealth.org/ Resources/Clinical-Care-Resources/Mental-Health/Mental-Health-Resources-For-Adolesc.aspx) offers a number of youth-friendly online mental-health resources.
- The American Academy of Pediatrics (AAP) has published guidance for clinicians on screening for emotional and behavioral disorders (pediatrics. aappublications.org/content/pediatrics/135/2/384.full.pdf).
- OAH has additional mental-health resources for professionals that are available in the TPP and PAF Resource Center (www.hhs.gov/ash/oah/ resources-and-training/tpp-and-paf-resources/index.html).
- SAMHSA's Suicide Prevention Resource Center (www.sprc.org) provides information on the role of high school teachers in preventing suicide.

Resources for Family Members

- The National Institute of Mental Health (NIMH) provides many resources, including a fact sheet on diagnosis and treatment for children with mental-health disorders (www.nimh.nih.gov/health/publications/treatment-of-children-with-mental-illness-fact-sheet/index.shtml).
- The Depression and Bipolar Support Alliance (DBSA) offers local support groups and online support groups for family members and friends of people with mental-health disorders.
- NAMI's Find Support section for families and caregivers (www.nami.org/ Find-Support/Family-Members-and-Caregivers) has guidance on what to do during a crisis, how to best support recovery, and taking care of your own

mental health. NAMI also runs support groups in communities around the country for family members.

- The HHS offers mental-health resources and information at MentalHealth.gov, including tips on how to talk to children about mental health (www.mentalhealth.gov/talk/parents-caregivers).

CHAPTER 47

LIFESTYLE MODIFICATIONS FOR MENTAL HEALTH AND WELL-BEING

About This Chapter: This chapter includes text excerpted from "Take Charge of Your Health: A Guide for Teenagers," National Institute of Diabetes and Digestive and Kidney Diseases (NIDDK), December 2016. Reviewed August 2020.

As you get older, you are able to start making your own decisions about a lot of things that matter most to you. You may choose your own clothes, music, and friends. You also may be ready to make decisions about your body and health. Making healthy decisions about what you eat and drink, how active you are, and how much sleep you get is a great place to start.

Do not forget to check out the "Did you know?" boxes for even more helpful tips and ideas.

How Does the Body Use Energy?

Your body needs energy to function and grow. Calories from food and drinks give you that energy. Think of food as energy to charge up your battery for the day. Throughout the day, you use energy from the battery to think and move, so you need to eat and drink to stay powered up. Balancing the energy you take in through food and beverages with the energy you use for growth, activity, and daily living is called "energy balance." Energy balance may help you stay a healthy weight.

How Many Calories Does Your Body Need?

Different people need different amounts of calories to be active or stay a healthy weight. The number of calories you need depends on whether you are male or female,

About 20 percent of kids between 12 and 19 years old have obesity. But, small changes in your eating and physical activity habits may help you reach and stay a healthy weight.

your genes, how old you are, your height and weight, whether you are still growing, and how active you are, which may not be the same every day.

How Should You Manage or Control Your Weight?

Some teens try to lose weight by eating very little; cutting out whole groups of foods like foods with carbohydrates, or "carbs;" skipping meals; or fasting. These approaches to losing weight could be unhealthy because they may leave out important nutrients your body needs. In fact, unhealthy dieting could get in the way of trying to manage your weight because it may lead to a cycle of eating very little and then overeating because you get too hungry. Unhealthy dieting could also affect your mood and how you grow.

Smoking, making yourself vomit, or using diet pills or laxatives to lose weight may also lead to health problems. If you make yourself vomit, or use diet pills or laxatives to control your weight, you could have signs of a serious eating disorder and should talk with your healthcare professional or another trusted adult right away. If you smoke, which increases your risk of heart disease, cancer, and other health problems, quit smoking as soon as possible.

If you think you need to lose weight, talk with a healthcare professional first. A doctor or dietitian may be able to tell you if you need to lose weight and how to do so in a healthy way.

Choose Healthy Foods and Drinks

Healthy eating involves taking control of how much and what types of food you eat, as well as the beverages you drink. Try to replace foods high in sugar, salt, and unhealthy fats with fruits, vegetables, whole grains, low-fat protein foods, and fat-free or low-fat dairy foods.

Fruits and Vegetables

Make half of your plate fruits and vegetables. Dark green, red, and orange vegetables have high levels of the nutrients you need, like vitamin C, calcium, and fiber. Adding tomato and spinach—or any other available greens that you like—to your sandwich is an easy way to get more veggies in your meal.

Grains

Choose whole grains like whole-wheat bread, brown rice, oatmeal, and whole-grain cereal, instead of refined-grain cereals, white bread, and white rice.

Protein

Power up with low fat or lean meats like turkey or chicken, and other protein-rich foods, such as seafood, egg whites, beans, nuts, and tofu.

Dairy

Build strong bones with fat-free or low-fat milk products. If you cannot digest lactose—the sugar in milk that can cause stomach pain or gas—choose lactose-free milk

> **Healthy Eating Tips**
> - Try to limit foods like cookies, candy, frozen desserts, chips, and fries, which often have a lot of sugar, unhealthy fat, and salt.
> - For a quick snack, try recharging with a pear, apple, or banana; a small bag of baby carrots; or hummus with sliced veggies.
> - Do not add sugar to your food and drinks.
> - Drink fat-free or low-fat milk and avoid sugary drinks. Soda, energy drinks, sweet tea, and some juices have added sugars, a source of extra calories. The *2015–2020 Dietary Guidelines* (health.gov/our-work/food-nutrition/2015-2020-dietary-guidelines/guidelines/executive-summary) call for getting less than 10 percent of your daily calories from added sugars.

or soy milk with added calcium. Fat-free or low-fat yogurt is also a good source of dairy food.

Fats

Fat is an important part of your diet. Fat helps your body grow and develop, and may even keep your skin and hair healthy. But, fats have more calories per gram than protein or carbs, and some are not healthy.

Some fats, such as oils that come from plants and are liquid at room temperature, are better for you than other fats. Foods that contain healthy oils include avocados, olives, nuts, seeds, and seafood such as salmon and tuna fish.

Solid fats such as butter, stick margarine, and lard, are solid at room temperature. These fats often contain saturated and trans fats, which are not healthy for you. Other foods with saturated fats include fatty meats, and cheese and other dairy products made from whole milk. Take it easy on foods like fried chicken, cheeseburgers, and fries, which often have a lot of saturated and trans fats. Options to consider include a turkey sandwich with mustard or a lean-meat, turkey, or veggie burger.

Your body needs a small amount of sodium, which is mostly found in salt. But, getting too much sodium from your foods and drinks can raise your blood pressure, which is unhealthy for your heart and your body in general. Even though you are a teen, it is important to pay attention to your blood pressure and heart health now to prevent health problems as you get older.

Try to consume less than 2,300 mg, or no more than 1 teaspoon, of sodium a day. This amount includes the salt in already prepared food, as well as the salt you add when cooking or eating your food.

Processed foods, like those that are canned or packaged, often have more sodium than unprocessed foods, such as fresh fruits and vegetables. When you can, choose fresh or frozen fruits and veggies over processed foods. Try adding herbs and spices instead of salt to season your food if you make your own meals. Remember to rinse canned vegetables with water to remove extra salt. If you use packaged foods,

Did You Know?

Many teens need more of these nutrients:

- Calcium, to build strong bones and teeth. Good sources of calcium are fat-free or low-fat milk, yogurt, and cheese.
- Vitamin D, to keep bones healthy. Good sources of vitamin D include orange juice, whole oranges, tuna, and fat-free or low-fat milk.
- Potassium, to help lower blood pressure. Try a banana, or baked potato with the skin, for a potassium boost.
- Fiber, to help you stay regular and feel full. Good sources of fiber include beans and celery.
- Protein, to power you up and help you grow strong. Peanut butter; eggs; tofu; legumes, such as lentils and peas; and chicken, fish, and low-fat meats are all good sources of protein.
- Iron, to help you grow. Red meat contains a form of iron that your body absorbs best. Spinach, beans, peas, and iron-fortified cereals are also sources of iron. You can help your body absorb the iron from these foods better when you also eat foods with vitamin C, like an orange.

check the amount of sodium listed on the Nutrition Facts label (www.fda.gov/food/nutrition-education-resources-materials/new-nutrition-facts-label).

Limit Added Sugars

Some foods, like fruit, are naturally sweet. Other foods, like ice cream and baked desserts, as well as some beverages, have added sugars to make them taste sweet. These sugars add calories, but not vitamins or fiber. Try to consume less than 10 percent of your daily calories from added sugars in food and beverages. Reach for an apple or banana instead of a candy bar.

Control Your Food Portions

A portion is how much food or beverage you choose to consume at one time, whether in a restaurant, from a package, at school or a friend's, or at home. Many people consume larger portions than they need, especially when away from home. Ready-to-eat meals—from a restaurant, grocery store, or at school—may give you larger portions than your body needs to stay charged up. Follow these tips to help you eat and drink a suitable amount of food and beverages, whether you are at home or somewhere else.

Do Not Skip Meals

Skipping meals might seem like an easy way to lose weight, but it actually may lead to weight gain if you eat more later to make up for it. Even if you are really busy with school and activities, it is important to try not to skip meals. Follow these tips to keep your body charged up all day and to stay healthy:

- Eat breakfast every day. Breakfast helps your body get going. If you are short on time in the morning, grab something to go, like an apple or banana.

Did You Know?

Just one super-sized, fast food meal may have more calories than you need in a whole day. And when people are served more food, they may eat or drink more—even if they do not need it. This habit may lead to weight gain. When consuming fast food, choose small portions or healthier options, like a veggie wrap or salad instead of fries or fried chicken.

Be Media Smart

Advertisements, TV shows, the Internet, and social media may affect your food and beverage choices and how you choose to spend your time. Many ads try to get you to consume high-fat foods and sugary drinks. Be aware of some of the tricks ads use to influence you:

- An ad may show a group of teens consuming a food or drink, or using a product to make you think all teens are or should be doing the same. The ad may even use phrases like "all teens need" or "all teens are."
- Advertisers sometimes show famous people using or recommending a product because they think you will want to buy products that your favorite celebrities use.
- Ads often use cartoon figures to make a food, beverage, or activity look exciting and appealing to young people.

- Pack your lunch on school days. Packing your lunch may help you control your food and beverage portions and increases the chances that you will eat it because you made it.
- Eat dinner with your family. When you eat home-cooked meals with your family, you are more likely to consume healthy foods. Having meals together also gives you a chance to reconnect with each other and share news about your day.
- Get involved in grocery shopping and meal planning at home. Going food shopping and planning and preparing meals with family members or friends can be fun. Not only can you choose a favorite grocery store, and healthy foods and recipes, you also have a chance to help others in your family eat healthy too.

Did You Know?

Teens who eat breakfast may do better in school. By eating breakfast, you can increase your memory and stay focused during the school day.

Get Moving

Physical activity should be part of your daily life, whether you play sports, take physical education (PE) classes in school, do chores, or get around by biking or walking. Regular physical activity can help you manage your weight, have stronger muscles and bones, and be more flexible.

Aerobic versus Lifestyle Activities

You should be physically active for at least 60 minutes a day. Most of the 60 minutes or more of activity a day should be either moderate- or vigorous-intensity aerobic physical activity, and you should include vigorous-intensity physical activity at least 3 days a week. Examples of aerobic physical activity, or activity that makes you breathe harder and speeds up your heart rate, include jogging, biking, and dancing.

For a more moderate workout, try brisk walking, jogging, or biking on flat streets or paths. To pick up the intensity, turn your walk into a jog, or your jog into a run—or add hills to your walk, jog, or bike ride. You do not have to do your 60 minutes a day all at once to benefit from your activity.

As part of your 60 minutes or more of daily physical activity, you should include muscle-strengthening physical activities, like lifting weights, on at least 3 days a week.

Routine activities, such as cleaning your room or taking out the trash, may not get your heart rate up the way biking or jogging does. But, they are also good ways to keep active on a regular basis.

Fitness apps that you can download onto your computer, smartphone, or other mobile device can help you keep track of how active you are each day.

Have Fun with Your Friends

Being active can be more fun with other people, like friends or family members. You may also find that you make friends when you get active by joining a sports team or dance club. Mix things up by choosing a different activity each day. Try kickball, flashlight tag, or other activities that get you moving, like walking around the mall. Involve

What If You Do Not Have Money for Sports Equipment or Activities?

You do not need money or equipment to stay active. You can run or use free community facilities, like school tracks and basketball courts, to be active at least 60 minutes each day. If you want to play a sport or game that you need equipment for, check with your neighbors or friends at school to see if you can borrow or share supplies. Your school guidance counselor or a PE teacher or coach could tell you how much it costs to join a sports team you are interested in. They may know if your school waived or reduced fees, or if you could apply for a "scholarship" for certain activities.

Tips for Cutting Back Your Screen Time

Try to limit your screen time to less than 2 hours each day, not counting your homework:
- Replace after-school TV and video-game time with physical activities at home, at school, or in your community.
- Turn off your cellphone or other device before you go to bed. Put them away from your nightstand or bed.

your friends and challenge them to be healthy with you. Sign up for active events together, like charity walks, fun runs, or scavenger hunts.

Take It Outside

Maybe you or some of your friends spend a lot of time indoors watching TV, surfing the web, using social media, or playing video games. Try getting in some outdoor activity to burn calories instead. Here are other activities to try:
- Have a jump rope or hula hoop contest.
- Play Frisbee.
- Build an obstacle course or have a scavenger hunt.
- Play volleyball or flag football.

If you are stuck indoors or do not have a lot of time, try climbing up and down the stairs in your apartment or home. You can also find dance and other fitness and exercise videos online or on some TV channels. Some routines are only 15 or 20 minutes so you can squeeze them in between homework, going out, or other activities. You also can choose active sports games if you have a gaming system.

Get Enough Sleep

Sometimes it is hard to get enough sleep, especially if you have a job, help take care of younger brothers or sisters, or are busy with other activities after school. Like healthy eating and getting enough physical activity, getting enough sleep is important for staying healthy.

You need enough sleep to do well in school, work and drive safely, and fight off infection. Not getting enough sleep may make you moody and irritable. While more research is needed, some studies have shown that not getting enough sleep may also contribute to weight gain.

If you are between 13 and 18 years old, you should get 8 to 10 hours of sleep each night.

Take Your Time

Changing your habits can be hard. And developing new habits takes time. Use the tips below and the checklist under "Be a health champion" to stay motivated and meet your goals. You can do it!

- **Make changes slowly.** Do not expect to change your eating, drinking, or activity habits overnight. Changing too much too fast may hurt your chances of success.
- **Figure out what is holding you back.** Are there unhealthy snack foods at home that are too tempting? Are the foods and drinks you are choosing at your school cafeteria too high in fat and sugar? How can you change these habits?
- **Set a few realistic goals.** If you are a soda drinker, try replacing a couple of sodas with water. Once you are drinking less soda for a while, try cutting out all soda. Then set another goal, like getting more physical activity each day. Once you have reached one goal, add another.
- **Get a buddy at school or someone at home to support your new habits.** Ask a friend, brother or sister, parent, or guardian to help you make changes and stick with your new habits.

Planning Healthy Meals and Physical Activities Just for You

Being healthy sounds like it could be a lot of work, right? Well, it does not have to be. A free, online tool called the "MyPlate Daily Checklist" (www.choosemyplate.gov/widgets-sm/myplate-plan-start) can help you create a daily food plan. All you have to do is type in whether you are male or female, your weight, height, and how much physical activity you get each day. The checklist will tell you how many daily calories you should take in and what amounts of fruit, vegetables, grains, protein, and dairy you should eat to stay within your calorie target.

Another tool, called the "NIH Body Weight Planner (www.niddk.nih.gov/health-information/weight-management/body-weight-planner)" lets you tailor your calorie and physical activity plans to reach your personal goals within a specific time period.

For recipes to help you plan easy and healthy meals like the ones below, visit BAM! Body and Mind (www.cdc.gov/healthyschools/bam/teachers.htm).

Breakfast: a banana, a slice of whole-grain bread with avocado or tomato, and fat-free or low-fat milk

Lunch: a turkey sandwich with dark leafy lettuce, tomato, and red peppers on whole-wheat bread

Dinner: two whole-grain taco shells with chicken or black beans, fat-free or low-fat cheese, and romaine lettuce

Snack: an apple, banana, or air-popped popcorn

Be a Health Champion

Spending much of your day away from home can sometimes make it hard to consume healthy foods and drinks. By becoming a "health champion," you can help yourself and family members, as well as your friends, get healthier by consuming healthier foods and drinks and becoming more active. Use this checklist to work healthy habits into your day, whether you are at home or on the go:

- Each night, pack a healthy lunch and snacks for the next day. Consume the lunch you packed. Try to avoid soda, chips, and candy from vending machines.
- Go to bed at a regular time every night to recharge your body and mind. Turn off your phone, TV, and other devices when you go to bed. Try to get between 8 and 10 hours of sleep each night.
- Eat a healthy breakfast.
- Walk or bike to school if you live nearby and can do so safely. Invite friends to join you.
- Between classes, stand up and walk around, even if your next subject is in the same room.
- Participate in gym classes instead of sitting on the sidelines.
- Get involved in choosing food and drinks at home. Help make dinner and share it with your family at the dinner table.

CHAPTER 48
CONTROLLING VAPE CRAVINGS TRIGGERED BY ANXIETY OR DEPRESSION

About This Chapter: Text beginning with the heading "Anxiety, Stress, and Vaping" is excerpted from "Anxiety, Stress, and Vaping," Smokefree Teen, U.S. Department of Health and Human Services (HHS), July 19, 2019; Text under the heading "Depression and Vaping" is excerpted from "Depression and Vaping," Smokefree Teen, U.S. Department of Health and Human Services (HHS), July 19, 2019.

Anxiety, Stress, and Vaping

Stress is a normal part of life—everyday worries, responsibilities, and hassles all contribute to your overall stress level. Too much stress can make you feel overwhelmed and affect your mood. If you automatically reach for your vape when you are stressed out try creating a personalized quit plan to help you come up with strategies for dealing with stress without vaping.

Anxiety is feeling worried, nervous, or panicky. Anxiety can be a reaction to stress, or it can be triggered by other things in your life. It is normal to experience anxiety from time to time—but anxiety can be a problem if it is frequent or interferes with your daily life.

Even if you rarely felt stressed or anxious before quitting vaping, you may feel increased stress, irritability or anxiety after quitting. For some people, the experience of quitting can feel overwhelming. It might be hard to imagine yourself or your life without your vape. The good news is that these mood changes are usually temporary while your body adjusts to being without nicotine. The longer you go without nicotine, the better you will feel. When you are having a rough day, remember why quitting vaping will be better for you in the long run.

Tips for Managing Stress and Anxiety

Stress and anxiety can trigger vape cravings, and make it harder for you to quit for good. You may be tempted to reach for your vape when you have these feelings, but vaping is not an effective way to cope. There are healthy and effective ways to deal with stress and anxiety.

Stop and Breathe

Pause what you are doing, and take a deep breath in through your nose and out through your mouth. Concentrate on the inhale and the exhale of your breath. Interrupting the anxious feeling with conscious breathing can help you calm down and think clearly.

Learn Your Anxiety Triggers

Anxiety can happen without being triggered. But, certain people, places, and situations can also trigger anxiety. Identify what makes you feel anxious or panicked and record it on your phone or in a journal. Do you see a pattern? Understanding your triggers is the first step in learning how to manage them.

Move Your Body

Getting your body moving is a great way to reduce stress and anxiety. When you exercise, your brain releases chemicals that make you feel good. Take a walk, hit the gym, or do some yoga.

Care for Yourself

Eating a balanced diet, drinking lots of water, and getting enough sleep will help your body keep your stress level down. Keep healthy snacks on hand, and do not skip meals.

Be Present

Life can be overwhelming, especially when you get caught up in worrying about what is next. Instead, focus on what you can control and try to stay in the moment.

Decaffeinate

Caffeine can help you stay awake, but it can also make you feel tense, jittery, and stressed. That is not helpful when you are quitting vaping. Cutting back on or gradually eliminating caffeinated products—like coffee, energy drinks, and some sodas—while you are quitting can reduce feelings of stress and anxiety.

Reach Out to Loved Ones

You do not have to deal with stress alone. Focus on spending time with people who make you feel good about yourself and want to help you stay vape-free. Talk to your friends, family, teachers, school counselors, and other important people in your life who support you and your decision to stop vaping.

Accept Life's Ups and Downs

Life is full of twists and turns. You will always have some stress in your life. It helps to understand that there will be good days and bad days.

Look Out for Signs of Serious Anxiety

Feeling anxious or irritable as you are quitting vaping is normal. But if you are feeling extreme anxiety or mood changes, you may need help from a professional. You may feel like the symptoms are too extreme or would not go away. Watch for this, especially if you have ever had severe anxiety. If you feel like the anxiety is overwhelming, tell a supportive friend or family member, and talk to your doctor.

Depression and Vaping

Sadness is a common emotion that can be triggered by ordinary life circumstances like disappointments, challenges, or loss. Everyone has down days and times when they feel sad. If feelings of sadness are extreme, last for a long time, or interfere with your daily activities and/or relationships, you may be experiencing a depressed mood.

Even if you rarely felt sad before quitting vaping, you may feel increased sadness, irritability or sluggishness after quitting. These mood changes are usually temporary while your body adjusts to being without nicotine. When you are having a rough day, remember why quitting vaping will be better for you in the long run.

You can learn to manage your feelings without reaching for your vape. Try these ideas—some may work better than others, so find the ones that work for you.

Get Active

Any kind of physical activity can help boost your mood. For example, taking a walk, going to the gym, or playing Frisbee with friends. If you need to, start small and build up over time. This can be hard to do because feeling down can drain your energy, but making the effort will pay off. It will help you feel better in the long run.

Stay Busy

Sadness and negative thoughts tend to creep up when you are bored and doing nothing. Create a schedule of activities that you will do every day. Sticking to a daily routine can help you stay busy and avoid getting caught up in negative moods.

Do Something You Enjoy Each Day

Find ways to incorporate fun activities into your daily life. Small things—like watching your favorite show or listening to music—add up and can help your mood. Choose an activity that you really enjoy but have not done in a while, or try something new that you have always wanted to do.

Talk with Friends and Loved Ones

Getting support from the important people in your life can help your mood and make a big difference as you quit. They can be key to helping you feel better. Focus on spending time with people who make you feel good about yourself and want you to succeed in staying vape-free.

Do Good

Small acts of kindness, like letting someone else go ahead of you in line, picking up litter, or giving someone a compliment, can boost your mood.

Accept Life's Ups and Downs

Life is full of twists and turns. It helps to understand that there will be good days and bad days.

Look Out for Signs of Depression

It is normal to have ups and downs in your mood as you quit vaping. But if you are feeling extreme sadness or mood changes, you may need help from a mental-health professional. You may feel like the sadness is lasting too long or would not go away. Do not ignore these feelings, especially if a doctor has ever diagnosed you with depression. Take a quick quiz to find out if you have signs of depression. If you become depressed or are having extreme sadness, let a friend or family member know, and think about talking to your doctor.

CHAPTER 49
CUTTING BACK ON CAFFEINE

About This Chapter: Text beginning with the heading "What Is Caffeine?" is excerpted from "Caffeine," MedlinePlus, National Institutes of Health (NIH), April 14, 2020; Text under the heading "Tips to Avoid Caffeine" is excerpted from "The Buzz on Caffeine," National Institute on Drug Abuse (NIDA) for Teens, June 25, 2014. Reviewed August 2020.

What Is Caffeine?
Caffeine is a bitter substance that occurs naturally in more than 60 plants including:
- Coffee beans
- Tea leaves
- Kola nuts, which are used to flavor soft drink colas
- Cacao pods, which are used to make chocolate products

There is also synthetic (human-made) caffeine, which is added to some medicines, foods, and drinks. For example, some pain relievers, cold medicines, and over-the-counter (OTC) medicines for alertness contain synthetic caffeine. So do energy drinks and "energy-boosting" gums and snacks.

Most people consume caffeine from drinks. The amounts of caffeine in different drinks can vary a lot, but it is generally:
- An 8-ounce cup of coffee: 95–200 mg
- A 12-ounce can of cola: 35–45 mg
- An 8-ounce energy drink: 70–100 mg
- An 8-ounce cup of tea: 14–60 mg

What Are Caffeine's Effects on the Body?
Caffeine has many effects on your body's metabolism. It:
- Stimulates your central nervous system, which can make you feel more awake and give you a boost of energy
- Is a diuretic, meaning that it helps your body get rid of extra salt and water by urinating more

- Increases the release of acid in your stomach, sometimes leading to an upset stomach or heartburn
- May interfere with the absorption of calcium in the body
- Increases your blood pressure

Within one hour of eating or drinking caffeine, it reaches its peak level in your blood. You may continue to feel the effects of caffeine for four to six hours.

What Are the Side Effects from Too Much Caffeine?

For most people, it is not harmful to consume up to 400mg of caffeine a day. If you do eat or drink too much caffeine, it can cause health problems, such as:

- Restlessness and shakiness
- Insomnia
- Headaches
- Dizziness
- Rapid or abnormal heart rhythm
- Dehydration
- Anxiety
- Dependency, so you need to take more of it to get the same results

Some people are more sensitive to the effects of caffeine than others.

Who Should Avoid or Limit Caffeine?

You should check with your healthcare provider about whether you should limit or avoid caffeine if you:

- Are pregnant, since caffeine passes through the placenta to your baby
- Are breastfeeding, since a small amount of caffeine that you consume is passed along to your baby
- Have sleep disorders, including insomnia
- Have migraines or other chronic headaches
- Have anxiety
- Have gastroesophageal reflux disease (GERD) or ulcers
- Have fast or irregular heart rhythms
- Have high blood pressure
- Take certain medicines or supplements, including stimulants, certain antibiotics, asthma medicines, and heart medicines. Check with your healthcare provider about whether there might be interactions between caffeine and any medicines and supplements that you take.
- Are a child or teen. Neither should have as much caffeine as adults. Children can be especially sensitive to the effects of caffeine.

What Is Caffeine Withdrawal?

If you have been consuming caffeine on a regular basis and then suddenly stop, you may have caffeine withdrawal. Symptoms can include:

- Headaches
- Drowsiness
- Irritability
- Nausea
- Difficulty concentrating

These symptoms usually go away after a couple of days.

Tips to Avoid Caffeine

Drinking a cup of coffee, or eating a bar of chocolate, is usually not a big deal. But, there are alternatives to caffeine if you are looking for an energy burst but do not want to get that jittery feeling caffeine sometimes causes. Here are a few alternatives you can try to feel energized without overdoing the caffeine:

- **Sleep.** This may sound obvious, but getting enough sleep is important.
- **Eat regularly.** When you do not eat, your glucose (sugar) levels drop, making you feel drained. Some people find it helpful to eat four or five smaller meals throughout the day instead of fewer big meals.
- **Drink enough water.** Since our bodies are more than two-thirds H2O, we need at least 64 ounces of water a day.
- **Take a walk.** If you are feeling drained in the middle of the day, it helps to move around. Do sit-ups or jumping jacks. Go outside for a brisk walk or ride your bike.

CHAPTER 50

ACADEMIC ACCOMMODATIONS FOR STUDENTS WITH PSYCHIATRIC DISABILITY

About This Chapter: This chapter includes text excerpted from "Mental Health on College Campuses: Investments, Accommodations Needed to Address Student Needs," National Council on Disability (NCD), July 21, 2017.

Reasonable Modifications and Accommodations

Under the Americans with Disabilities Act (ADA) and Section 504, colleges must provide students with disabilities reasonable modifications to their policies, practices, and procedures unless doing so would fundamentally alter the nature of its service, program, or activity. Modifications are made on a case-by-case basis. Colleges should, however, have reasonable modification policies in place and ensure that all staff who work with students receive training on those policies. Colleges should ensure that students have access to those policies as well. The University of Washington is a good example of how a college can share information about modifications/accommodations for students with disabilities via the college website. Reasonable modifications may include flexible class and/or attendance schedules, leave of absence (LOAs) without financial penalties, and other changes to standard policies that allow students with mental-health disabilities to remain in, and succeed in, college.

Most Important Accommodations for Students with Mental-Health Disabilities

- Excused absences for treatment (54%)
- Medical leaves of absence and course withdrawals without penalty (46%)
- Adjustments in test settings (34%)
- Homework deadline extensions and adjustments in test times (33%)
- Increased availability of academic advisors (32%)

In addition, the Fair Housing Act (FHA) and Section 504 require colleges to allow students with mental-health disabilities who require an emotional support animal to keep such animals in college housing as a reasonable accommodation.

According to the National Alliance on Mental Illness (NAMI) survey, 62 percent of students said they knew how to access accommodations, and 43 percent did access them. Students reported that their most important accommodations were excused absences for treatment (54%), medical LOAs and course withdrawals without penalty (46%), adjustments in test settings (34%), homework deadline extensions and adjustments in test times (33%), and increased availability of academic advisors (32%).

Ten percent of the practitioner questionnaire respondents reported that institutional bias could be creating barriers to mental-health services and supports. Some believed lack of training for faculty allowed some students to slip through the cracks. One respondent noted that there is likely "some institutional cultural bias that colleges should not be providing health services to student's and/or a reluctance to promote service availability" that helps lead to barriers that keep students away.

Because mental-health disabilities are invisible, students often find themselves trying to negotiate accommodations with faculty members who do not understand their disability-related needs. Students must be diagnosed with a disability to request reasonable modifications/ accommodations, as students without a verified disability are not covered by the ADA, Section 504, or the FHA. Faculty who have not received training can be resistant to making "exceptions," especially for "invisible" disabilities, even when appropriate disability verification is in place. This finding relates to previous findings from both practitioners and students that faculty need more training in disability-related accommodations.

CHAPTER 51

WORKPLACE ACCOMMODATIONS FOR YOUTH WITH MENTAL-HEALTH NEEDS

About This Chapter: This chapter includes text excerpted from "Entering the World of Work: What Youth with Mental Health Needs Should Know about Accommodations," Office of Disability Employment Policy (ODEP), U.S. Department of Labor (DOL), April 11, 2007. Reviewed August 2020.

Starting a job can be difficult for any young person. If you happen to have a hidden disability, such as a mental-health impairment, a new workplace can be overwhelming. If you have ever felt this way, you are not alone. According to the National Institute of Mental Health (NIMH), the leading cause of disability in the United States for ages 15 to 44 is major depressive disorder (and this is only one type of mental-health impairment). Along with questions about the job itself, you may have questions about when and how to disclose your disability. You may wonder if it is appropriate to ask for modifications in your new work setting. This chapter provides guidance to assist you with a successful transition into the workforce by answering questions regarding disclosure, accommodations, and resources.

Requesting an Accommodation

Many employers are aware of accommodations for people with physical disabilities, but may not know how to accommodate people with invisible disabilities. Unlike in high school, it is your responsibility to ask for accommodation. You need to be aware of your individual needs and abilities and be able to communicate them to your employer.

People with disabilities can request an accommodation at any time during the application process or while employed. To request an accommodation, you have to inform your employer of the need for an adjustment or change at work for a reason related to your disability. There are no keywords you must use in order to make the request, and neither the Americans with Disabilities Act (ADA) nor the phrase "reasonable accommodation" has to be mentioned. Do not be afraid to ask your employer for a work-related accommodation if it will help you perform your job better.

Table 51.1. Some Common Types of Reasonable Accommodations

Challenge	Possible Accommodations
Maintaining consistent attendance	• Flexible leave to attend counseling • Making up time missed • Schedule a later start time
Dealing with change	• Maintaining open lines of communication with supervisor • Scheduling regular meetings with supervisor to discuss work-related issues
Interacting with others	• Providing a mentor, a team leader or a buddy to facilitate social and work-related interactions • Participating in team activities
Managing time	• An electronic calendar marked with meetings and deadlines • Use e-mail as a time management tool • Daily or weekly performance goals • A partner or a mentor to help with time management
Organizing information	• Assistance in prioritizing tasks • A written to-do list, which can be reviewed on a regular basis • Dividing large assignments into smaller tasks • A personal data assistant or other electronic organizer
Handling stress and emotions	• Short breaks to walk around the block • Praise and positive reinforcement • Permission to call or instant message a support person
Maintaining concentration	• A quiet location • Space enclosures • Wearing a headset or ear sets and listening to music or "white noise"

Some Common Types of Reasonable Accommodations

Below are some common challenges and possible accommodations you might ask your employer to consider. If you decide to disclose your disability and ask your employer for an accommodation, it is a good idea to have already considered what type of accommodation you need to better perform your job. This list may help you think about possible solutions.

PART 6 | IF YOU NEED MORE HELP OR INFORMATION

CHAPTER 52

DIRECTORY OF ORGANIZATIONS THAT HELP PEOPLE WITH ANXIETY, DEPRESSION, AND OTHER MENTAL-HEALTH CONCERNS

About This Chapter: Resources in this chapter were compiled from several sources deemed reliable; all contact information was verified and updated in August 2020.

Government Agencies That Provide Information about Anxiety and Depression

Agency for Healthcare Research and Quality (AHRQ)
5600 Fishers Ln.
Rockville, MD 20857
Phone: 301-427-1104
Website: www.ahrq.gov

Centers for Disease Control and Prevention (CDC)
1600 Clifton Rd.
Atlanta, GA 30329-4027
Toll-Free: 800-CDC-INFO (800-232-4636)
Phone: 404-639-3311
Toll-Free TTY: 888-232-6348
Website: www.cdc.gov
E-mail: cdcinfo@cdc.gov

Child Welfare Information Gateway

United States Children's Bureau
330 C St. S.W.
Washington, DC 20201
Toll-Free: 800-394-3366
Website: www.childwelfare.gov
E-mail: info@childwelfare.gov

MedlinePlus

National Institutes of Health (NIH)
8600 Rockville Pike
Bethesda, MD 20894
Toll-Free: 888-FIND-NLM (888-346-3656)
Phone: 301-594-5983
Website: www.medlineplus.gov

MentalHealth.gov

U.S. Department of Health and Human Services (HHS)
200 Independence Ave. S.W.
Washington, DC 20201
Website: www.mentalhealth.gov

National Center for Complementary and Integrative Health (NCCIH)

9000 Rockville Pike
Bethesda, MD 20892
Toll-Free: 888-644-6226
Toll-Free TTY: 866-464-3615
Website: www.nccih.nih.gov
E-mail: info@nccih.nih.gov

National Institute of Diabetes and Digestive and Kidney Diseases (NIDDK)

9000 Rockville Pike
Bethesda, MD 20892
Toll-Free: 800-860-8747
Toll-Free TTY: 866-569-1162
Website: www.niddk.nih.gov
E-mail: healthinfo@niddk.nih.gov

National Institute of Food and Agriculture (NIFA)

U.S. Department of Agriculture (USDA)
1400 Independence Ave. S.W.
Stop 2201
Washington, DC 20250-2201
Website: nifa.usda.gov

National Institute of Mental Health (NIMH)

Office of Science Policy, Planning, and Communications (OSPPC)
6001 Executive Blvd.
Rm. 6200, MSC 9663
Bethesda, MD 20892-9663
Toll-Free: 866-615-NIMH (866-615-6464)
Toll-Free TTY: 866-415-8051
TTY: 301-443-8431
Fax: 301-443-4279
Website: www.nimh.nih.gov
E-mail: nimhinfo@nih.gov

National Institute on Aging (NIA)

31 Center Dr., MSC 2292
Bldg. 31, Rm. 5C27
Bethesda, MD 20892
Toll-Free: 800-222-2225
Toll-Free TTY: 800-222-4225
Website: www.nia.nih.gov
E-mail: niaic@nia.nih.gov

National Institute on Drug Abuse (NIDA)

Office of Science Policy and Communications (OSPC)
6001 Executive Blvd.
Rm. 5213, MSC 9561
Bethesda, MD 20892
Phone: 301-443-1124
Website: www.drugabuse.gov

National Institutes of Health (NIH)

9000 Rockville Pike
Bethesda, MD 20892
Phone: 301-496-4000
TTY: 301-402-9612
Website: www.nih.gov

NIH News in Health

NIH Office of Communications and Public Liaison (OCPL)
Bldg. 31
Rm. 5B52
Bethesda, MD 20892-2094
Phone: 301-451-8224
Website: newsinhealth.nih.gov
E-mail: nihnewsinhealth@od.nih.gov

StopBullying.gov

U.S. Department of Health and Human Services (HHS)
200 Independence Ave. S.W.
Washington, DC 20201
Website: www.stopbullying.gov

Substance Abuse and Mental Health Services Administration (SAMHSA)

5600 Fishers Ln.
Rockville, MD 20857
Toll-Free: 877-SAMHSA-7 (877-726-4727)
Toll-Free TTY: 800-487-4889
Website: www.samhsa.gov
E-mail: samhsainfo@samhsa.hhs.gov

U.S. Department of Health and Human Services (HHS)

200 Independence Ave. S.W.
Washington, DC 20201
Toll-Free: 877-696-6775
Website: www.hhs.gov

U.S. Department of Labor (DOL)

200 Constitution Ave. N.W.
Washington, DC 20210
Toll-Free: 866-4-USA-DOL (866-487-2365)
Website: www.dol.gov

U.S. Department of Veterans Affairs (VA)

Toll-Free: 844-698-2311
Toll-Free TTY: 844-698-2711
Website: www.va.gov

U.S. Food and Drug Administration (FDA)

10903 New Hampshire Ave.
Silver Spring, MD 20993-0002
Toll-Free: 888-INFO-FDA (888-463-6332)
Website: www.fda.gov

Youth.gov

Toll-Free: 877-231-7843
Website: www.youth.gov
E-mail: youthgov@air.org

Private Agencies That Provide Information about Anxiety and Depression

Active Minds

2001 S. St. N.W.
Ste. 630
Washington, DC 20009
Phone: 202-332-9595
Fax: 202-332-9599
Website: www.activeminds.org

Alzheimer's Foundation of America

322 Eighth Ave.
16th Fl.
New York, NY 10001
Toll-Free: 866-232-8484
Website: www.alzfdn.org
E-mail: info@alzfdn.org

American Academy of Child and Adolescent Psychiatry (AACAP)

3615 Wisconsin Ave. N.W.
Washington, DC 20016-3007
Phone: 202-966-7300
Fax: 202-464-0131
Website: www.aacap.org

American Academy of Neurology (AAN)

201 Chicago Ave.
Minneapolis, MN 55415
Toll-Free: 800-879-1960
Phone: 612-928-6000
Fax: 612-454-2746
Website: www.aan.com
E-mail: memberservices@aan.com

American Association of Suicidology (AAS)

5221 Wisconsin Ave. N.W.
Second Fl.
Washington, DC 20015
Phone: 202-237-2280
Fax: 202-237-2282
Website: suicidology.org
E-mail: info@suicidology.org

American Bar Association (ABA)

321 N. Clark St.
Chicago, IL 60654
Toll-Free: 800-285-2221
Website: www.americanbar.org
E-mail: Service@americanbar.org

American Foundation for Suicide Prevention (AFSP)

199 Water St.
11th Fl.
New York, NY 10038
Toll-Free: 888-333-2377
Phone: 212-363-3500
Fax: 212-363-6237
Website: afsp.org
E-mail: info@afsp.org

American Medical Association (AMA)

AMA Plaza
330 N. Wabash Ave.
Ste. 39300
Chicago, IL 60611-5885
Toll-Free: 800-262-3211
Phone: 312-464-4782
Website: www.ama-assn.org

American Psychiatric Association Foundation (APA Foundation)

800 Maine Ave. S.W.
Ste. 900
Washington, DC 20024
Toll-Free: 888-357-7924
Phone: 202-559-3900
Website: www.psychiatry.org
E-mail: apa@psych.org

American Psychiatric Nurses Association (APNA)

3141 Fairview Park Dr., Ste. 625
Falls Church, VA 22042
Toll-Free: 855-863-APNA (855-863-2762)
Phone: 571-533-1919
Toll-Free Fax: 855-883-APNA (855-883-2762)
Website: www.apna.org
E-mail: inform@apna.org

Association for Behavioral Health & Wellness (ABHW)

1325 G St. N.W.
Ste. 500
Washington, DC 20005
Phone: 202-449-7660
Website: abhw.org
E-mail: info@abhw.org

Brain & Behavior Research Foundation

747 Third Ave.
33rd Fl.
New York, NY 10017
Toll-Free: 800-829-8289
Phone: 646-681-4888
Website: www.bbrfoundation.org
E-mail: info@bbrfoundation.org

Brain Trauma Foundation

228 Hamilton Ave.
Third Fl.
Palo Alto, CA 94301
Website: www.braintrauma.org

Child Mind Institute, Inc

101 E. 56th St.
New York, NY 10022
Phone: 212-308-3118
Website: childmind.org

Committee of Interns and Residents (CIR)/SEIU Healthcare

10-27 46th Ave., Ste. 300-2
Long Island City, NY 11101
Phone: 212-356-8100
Website: www.cirseiu.org
E-mail: info@cirseiu.org

Community Anti-Drug Coalitions of America (CADCA)

625 Slaters Ln.
Ste. 300
Alexandria, VA 22314
Toll-Free: 800-54-CADCA (800-542-2322)
Fax: 703-706-0565
Website: www.cadca.org

Families for Depression Awareness

391 Totten Pond Rd.
Ste. 101
Waltham, MA 02451
Phone: 781-890-0220
Fax: 781-890-2411
Website: www.familyaware.org
E-mail: info@familyaware.org

Family Caregiver Alliance® (FCA)

101 Montgomery St.
Ste. 2150
San Francisco, CA 94104
Toll-Free: 800-445-8106
Phone: 415-434-3388
Website: www.caregiver.org

International Foundation for Research and Education on Depression (iFred)

P.O. Box 17598
Baltimore, MD 21297
Fax: 443-782-0739
Website: www.ifred.org
E-mail: info@ifred.org

The Jed Foundation

6 E. 39th St.
Ste. 700
New York, NY 10016
Phone: 212-647-7544
Fax: 212-647-7542
Website: www.jedfoundation.org
E-mail: info@jedfoundation.org

Mental Health America (MHA)

500 Montgomery St.
Ste. 820
Alexandria, VA 22314
Toll-Free: 800-969-6642
Phone: 703-684-7722
Fax: 703-684-5968
Website: www.nmha.org
E-mail: info@mhanational.org

National Alliance on Mental Illness (NAMI)

4301 Wilson Blvd.
Ste. 300
Arlington, VA 22203
Toll-Free: 800-950-NAMI (800-950-6264)
Phone: 703-524-7600
Website: www.nami.org
E-mail: info@nami.org

National Association of County Behavioral Health and Developmental Disability Directors (NACBHDD)

660 N. Capitol St. N.W.
Ste. 400
Washington, DC 20001
Phone: 202-661-8816
Fax: 202-478-1659
Website: nacbhdd.org
E-mail: inquire@nacbhd.org

National Association of State Mental Health Program Directors (NASMHPD)

66 Canal Center Plaza
Ste. 302
Alexandria, VA 22314
Phone: 703-739-9333
Fax: 703-548-9517
Website: nasmhpd.org

National Child Traumatic Stress Network (NCTSN)

National Center for Child Traumatic Stress (NCCTS)
11150 W. Olympic Blvd.
Ste. 650
Los Angeles, CA 90064
Phone: 310-235-2633
Fax: 310-235-2612
Website: www.nctsn.org
E-mail: info@nctsn.org

National Coalition for Mental Health Recovery

2759 Martin Luther King, Jr. Ave. S.E.
Ste. 201
Washington, DC 20032
Phone: 202-642-4480
Website: www.ncmhr.org

National Council for Behavioral Health

1400 K St. N.W., Ste. 400
Washington, DC 20005
Phone: 202-684-7457
Website: www.thenationalcouncil.org

National Federation of Families for Children's Mental Health (NFFCMH)

15800 Crabbs Branch Way, Ste. 300
Rockville, MD 20855
Phone: 240-403-1901
Website: www.ffcmh.org
E-mail: ffcmh@ffcmh.org

National PTA

1250 N. Pitt St.
Alexandria, VA 22314
Toll Free: 800-307-4782
Phone: 703-518-1200
Fax: 703-836-0942
Website: www.pta.org
E-mail: info@pta.org

The Trevor Project

P.O. Box 69232
West Hollywood, CA 90069
Toll-Free: 866-488-7386
Phone: 310-271-8845
Website: www.thetrevorproject.org
E-mail: info@thetrevorproject.org

Youth M.O.V.E. National

P.O. Box 215
Decorah, IA 52101
Toll-Free: 800-580-6199
Website: youthmovenational.org
E-mail: info@youthmovenational.org

YWCA USA

1020 19th St. N.W., Ste. 750
Washington, DC 20036
Phone: 202-467-0801
Fax: 202-467-0802
Website: www.ywca.org
E-mail: info@ywca.org

INDEX

INDEX

Page numbers that appear in *Italics* refer to tables or illustrations. Page numbers that have a small 'n' after the page number refer to citation information shown as Notes. Page numbers that appear in **Bold** refer to information contained in boxes within the chapters.

APRN. *See* Advanced Practice Registered Nurse

aripiprazole, disruptive mood dysregulation disorder (DMDD), 71

ARNP. *See* Advanced Registered Nurse Practitioner

art and play therapy, overview, 119–20

ASD. *See* autism spectrum disorder

assertive community treatment (ACT), comorbid disorders treatment, 131

Association for Behavioral Health & Wellness (ABHW), contact, 241

asthma, caffeine, 226

attention deficit hyperactivity disorder (ADHD)
    brain circuits and mental disorders, 9
    children and mental health, 89
    common mental disorders, 13
    disruptive mood dysregulation disorder (DMDD), 70
    mental-health screening, 99

atypical antipsychotic, disruptive mood dysregulation disorder (DMDD), 71

AUD. *See* alcohol-use disorder

autism
    disruptive mood dysregulation disorder (DMDD), 71
    selective mutism (SM), 50

autism spectrum disorder (ASD), common mental disorders in young adults, 14

avoidance behavior
    agoraphobia, 59
    exposure therapy, 115

axon, brain circuits and mental disorders, 10

B

back pain, coping with stress, 175

BAI. *See* Beck Anxiety Inventory

BDI. *See* Beck Depression Inventory

Beck Anxiety Inventory (BAI), screening and diagnostic tools, 97

Beck Depression Inventory (BDI), screening and diagnostic tools, 98

Beck Hopelessness Scale, screening and diagnostic tools, 98

BED. *See* binge eating disorder

behavior problems
    protective and promotive factors in mental health, 154
    treating childhood depression, 103

behavioral health
    behavioral therapies, 131
    family therapy, 121
    mental health during COVID-19 pandemic, 208
    mental-health services, 191

behavioral therapy. *See* cognitive-behavioral therapy (CBT)

belly breathing, agoraphobia, 58

benzodiazepines
    agoraphobia, 59
    generalized anxiety disorder (GAD), 43
    panic disorders (PDs), 67

beta-blockers
    panic disorders (PDs), 67
    social anxiety disorder (SAD), 63

hiking, lifestyle modifications for mental health, 216

binge eating disorder (BED), common mental disorders in young adults, 14

bipolar disorder
    brain circuits and mental disorders, 9
    comorbid disorders treatment, 132
    mental-health myths and facts, 17
    screening for mental disorders, 100
    teen brain, 7
    See also manic depression

"black box" warning, disruptive mood dysregulation disorder (DMDD), 71

blood pressure
    brain circuits and mental disorders, 11
    caffeine, 226
    disruptive mood dysregulation disorder (DMDD), 71
    lifestyle modifications for mental health, 213

body image
    emotional and social development in adolescence, 147
    mental-health screening, 99

borderline personality disorder (BPD), comorbid disorders treatment, 131

BPD. *See* borderline personality disorder

brain
    anxiety disorders, 22
    childhood depression, 104
    common mental disorders in young adults, 15
    controlling vape cravings, 222
    emotional and social development in adolescence, 149
    generalized anxiety disorder (GAD), 42

I

IBD. *See* inflammatory bowel disease
illicit drugs
    anxiety disorders, 95, 107
    substance-use disorder (SUD), 14
illness management
    research grants, **143**
    supported care app, 141
imaginal exposure, defined, 116
immune system, toxic stress, 148
impulses
    brain growth, 7
    dendrites, 10
in vivo exposure
    agoraphobia, 58
    defined, 115
    See also cognitive-behavioral therapy (CBT)
incontinence, agoraphobia, 56
infections
    acupuncture, 133
    alcohol and drug use, 202
inflammatory bowel disease (IBD), cognitive-behavioral therapy (CBT), 135
injury
    bullying, 168
    mental-health problems, 18
    See also self-injury
insomnia
    antidepressant medicines, 112
    caffeine, 226
    DSM-5 criteria for depression, 97
    intervention apps, 142
    kava, 136
    psychotherapy, 108
    stimulant withdrawal, 85
    toxic stress, 148
Institute of Medicine (IOM), mental-health prevention, 37
insurance. *See* Children's Health Insurance Program (CHIP); health insurance
integrated group therapy (IGT), defined, 132
Interagency Working Group on Youth Programs (IWGYP), positive youth development, 36
International Foundation for Research and Education on Depression (iFred), contact, 242
Internet service providers (ISPs), cyberbullying, 169
interoceptive exposure
    defined, 116
    panic attacks, 58

intervention
    levels, depicted, 36
    mental-health disorder, 3, **143**
    mental-health evaluation, 90
    mental-health research, 15
    parent training, 71
    play therapy, 120
    selective mutism (SM), 51
    separation anxiety disorder (SAD), 47
    stress, 177
    substance-use disorders (SUDs), 128
    See also early intervention; psychosocial intervention
irrational fear. *See* phobia
irritability
    antidepressant, 27, 111
    anxiety disorder, 96
    caffeine withdrawal, 227
    disruptive mood dysregulation disorder (DMDD), 69
    lack of sleep, 8
    mental-health screening, 100
    premenstrual dysphoric disorder (PMDD), **79**
    vaping, 221
isolation
    panic disorder, 65
    social media, 186
    suicide risk, 202
    See also social isolation
ISPs. *See* Internet service providers

J

The Jed Foundation, contact, 242
job security
    generalized anxiety disorder (GAD), 42
    infectious disease outbreak, 203

K

KADS. *See* Kutcher Adolescent Depression Scale
kava, overview, 136–37
Kutcher Adolescent Depression Scale (KADS), depression, 98

L

lavender, anxiety, 137
laxatives
    eating disorder, 212
    student behavior, 199

psychotherapy
 anxiety disorders, 21
 cognitive-behavioral therapy (CBT), 131
 defined, 27, 43, 63, 71, 91
 mental-health problems, **3**
 relaxation techniques, 135
 See also cognitive-behavioral therapy; talk
  therapy
psychotic disorders, defined, 100
PTSD. *See* posttraumatic stress disorder
PTSD Symptom Scale—Self-Report Version,
 anxiety disorder screening, 97

Q

QOL. *See* quality of life
quality of life (QOL)
 disruptive mood dysregulation disorder
  (DMDD), 70
 helping individuals with mental-health
  problems, 19
 panic disorder (PD), 65
 separation anxiety disorder (SAD), 47
quarantine, COVID-19, 202

R

rapid or abnormal heart rhythm, caffeine, 226
reasonable accommodation, students with
 mental-health disabilities, 230
reassurance
 agoraphobia, 57
 attitudes and discrimination, 188
 children and mental health, 90
recovery
 agoraphobia, 57
 anxiety disorders treatment, 107
 attitudes and discrimination, 187
 behavioral health providers, 193
 childhood depression treatment, 105
 COVID-19, 207
 family therapy, 121
 integrated group therapy (IGT), 132
 people with mental-health problems, 18
 substance-induced depressive and anxiety
  disorder, 85
relapse
 antidepressant medications, 60
 childhood depression treatment, 104
 family therapy, 122
 integrated group therapy (IGT), 132

relationship
 adolescent mental health, 3
 behavioral health providers, 193
 children and mental health, 90
 depression and vaping, 223
 disruptive mood dysregulation disorder
  (DMDD), 70
 family therapy, 124
 generalized anxiety disorder (GAD), **42**
 importance of school connectedness, 161
 integrated group therapy (IGT), 132
 interpersonal therapy (IPT), 110
 multidimensional family therapy (MDFT), 128
 peer pressure, **172**
 positive youth development, 166
 protective and promotive factors in mental
  health, 154
 school-based mental-health services, 198
 treating anxiety in children, 120
 unique issues in emotional development, 148
relaxation
 agoraphobia, 57
 exposure therapy, 116
relaxation techniques
 described, 135
 exposure therapy, 117
 play therapy, 120
research
 adolescent friendship difficulties, 172
 brain regions, 11
 common mental-health disorders in
  adolescence, 15
 complementary approach, 135
 family therapy, 126
 generalized anxiety disorder (GAD), 42
 help-seeking attitude and reducing
  stigma, 186
 lifestyle modifications, 218
 panic disorder (PD), 66
 positive youth development, 165
 screening and diagnostic tools, 95
 selective mutism (SM), 51
 technology and mental-health treatment, 143
resilience
 anxiety disorders treatment, **108**
 protective and promotive factors in mental
  health, 153
 school-based mental-health support, 199
restless
 caffeine, 226